Do I Need to See the Doctor?
THE HOME TREATMENT ENCYCLOPEDIA
— WRITTEN BY MEDICAL DOCTORS — THAT LETS YOU DECIDE

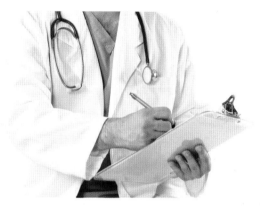

DR. BRIAN MURAT, DR. GREG STEWART and
DR. JOHN REA

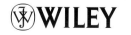WILEY

John Wiley & Sons Canada, Ltd.

Care has been taken to trace ownership of copyright material contained in this book. The publisher will gladly receive any information that will enable them to rectify any reference or credit line in subsequent editions.

Library and Archives Canada Cataloguing in Publication Data

Murat, Brian, 1960-

    Do I need to see the doctor? : the home-treatment encyclopedia, written by doctors, that lets you decide / Brian Murat, Greg Stewart, John Rea
Previous eds. published under title: Do I need to see the doctor? : a guide for treating common minor ailments at home for all ages.

ISBN 978-0-470-15972-9

1.   Self-care, Health. 2. Medicine, Popular-Encyclopedias. I. Stewart, Greg, 1960- II. Title.
2.   Rea, John, 1959-.
3.   RC81.M87 2008 616.02'4   C2008-905346-X

Production Credits
Photography: Ron Sumners © 2008
          Jenny Kirkpatrick © 2008 (pages 56, 61, 63, top 95, 149, 152)
Graphic Design: Ron Sumners, Sumners Graphics Inc.
Typesetting: Ron Sumners
Printer: Printcrafters

John Wiley & Sons Canada, Ltd.
6045 Freemont Blvd.
Mississauga, Ontario
L5R 4J3

Printed in Canada

1 2 3 4 5 PC 12 11 10 09 08

Attention

The approach to medical problems is always in evolution. The incorporation of new research, broader clinical knowledge, new technology and new medication may change the best way to manage medical problems. The writers, editors and publishers of this book have made their best effort to create a publication which uses the most up-to-date information available and have given advice that, at the time of publication, would be in accord with standards of practice. However, in view of human error, changes in medical science or misunderstanding by the reader, neither the writers, publishers nor any other party involved in the preparation or distribution of this publication warrants that information contained herein is in every respect accurate or complete, and they are not responsible for any errors or omissions or for the results obtained from use or misuse of such information. Readers are to be aware that this publication does not at any time replace medical practitioners and that people should always seek out a medical opinion if they feel it is warranted.

To our mothers

Whose practice of common sense home-based therapy is an inspiration. They swear that we are alive today as a direct result of their therapeutic application of a tincture of time, a mustard poultice or a gravol suppository whenever they were needed.

Table of contents

Acknowledgements

We would like to express our sincere thanks to the following individuals whose assistance in creating this book was invaluable.

Dr. Dann Morton
Dr. David Mathies
Dr. D. A. Jarvis
Dr. Derek Jones
Dr. Wendy Alexander
Dr. Su Sundaram
Victoria Mathies
Jane Withey
David Chilton
Bill Coon
Mary Jane Gordon
Donna Lynch
Dr. Peter White

The following Registered Trademarks are used in this publication and identified within using bold print.

Advil	Clearasil BP Plus	Maalox	Surfak
All Bran	Clearasil Stayclear	Metamucil	Tagament
Allegra	Cliniderm Soothing Lotion	Midol	Tamiflu
Aspirin	Colace	Milk of Magnesia	Tavist
Atrovent	Conestin	Motrin	Telfa
Auralgan	Correctol	Opticrom	Tempra
Axid	Depends	Oxy Daily	Triaminic
Bactine	Dimetane	Oxy 5	Tums
Benadryl	Dimetapp	Pedialyte	Tylenol
Benzagel	Dulcolax	Peniten	Valium
Biaxin	Exlax	Pepcid	Vaseline
Bran Buds	Fleet	Peptobismol	Vasocon
Bricanyl	Gastrolyte	Polysporin	Ventolin
Buro-sol	Gaviscon	Prepulsid	Viagra
Champix	Gravol	Prodiem	Visine
Chloraseptic	Hismanal	Riopan	Wild Strawberry
Chlor-Tripolon	Imodium	Rolaids	Zantac
Claritin	Kaopectate	Salinex	Zincofax
Clean and Clear	Kool-Aid	Sennakot	Zyban
Continuous Control	Lansoyl	Solarcaine	

The recommendation by the authors to use specifically named products in this publication is based solely on the authors' practice patterns. The list in no way represents the entire range of products available, nor does it suggest superiority over other products on the market. The authors recommend that consumers ask their pharmacists for advice about product purchases.

FOREWORD

The rationale for this invaluable publication is simple: it is satisfying to assist families in making independent decisions when caring for themselves, elderly relatives or sick infants. No one wants the inconvenience or worry of waiting to see the doctor if they do not need to. Making decisions for oneself is a wonderful, empowering feeling, and this little book can safely guide at a time when parents are anxious about a new infant or are faced with a sick child or elderly relative. Parents can, and should, trust their instincts about their own children and will find here the support they need. There is practical advice for the new mother struggling with her body's adjustments to childbirth, and for both parents, worried and exhausted, pacing with a crying baby in the wee hours of the morning, there is the answer to the common question, Is it safe to wait?

Do I Need to See the Doctor? is an excellent addition to the self-care library. Ever since John Wesley, the founder of the Methodist church, wrote his book, *Primitive Remedies*, in 1747, there have been scores of books published with the same intent. The uniqueness of this particular addition lies in its simplicity. Today, the ease of access to information on the Internet has given rise to a need for the simplification of information in one place. Not all home remedies are worthwhile, and people need to be able to trust what they are reading. The format of carefully researched flowcharts and authoritative and experienced advice ensures that trust. By necessity, this is not a comprehensive encyclopedia, but it is an important resource for the most common health problems for which patients seek guidance.

For the past several years, I have been privileged to be part of the discussions swirling around the need to deliver primary care to Canadians in a more effective yet comprehensive manner. It is evident that family physicians are not just a resource to their patients, but to the larger community as well. Encouraging parental and patient confidence, Drs. Murat, Stewart and Rea have contributed to the healthcare system well beyond their office walls. Resources like this, when used effectively, can improve access to care for all, since only those who really need medical attention seek it out. With healthcare resources stretched to the limit, any safe and effective way to reduce and streamline demands—such as this book—will be welcomed by healthcare providers and taxpayers alike. In fact, I think it would be a good idea for physicians to keep copies of *Do I Need to See the Doctor?* in their examination rooms, the better able to demonstrate to patients how to use this tool the next time similar symptoms develop.

David J. Mathies, MD, CCFP, FCFP
Past President, Ontario College of Family Physicians
Chief of Staff, Muskoka Algonquin Healthcare
Family Physician, Huntsville, Ontario

The Family Medicine Chest

Illnesses and accidents don't happen on a schedule. We suggest that you plan ahead and have the following products in your home for quick treatment without delay.

Acetaminophen (**Tylenol, Tempra** or generic)
in liquid, chewable tablets or regular tablet form as
appropriate for age. Check the dosage chart on page 58
to help you decide the dosage you need.

Ibuprofen (**Advil, Motrin** and others)
in tablet or liquid form for adult or child use

Dimetapp or other combination
decongestant and antihistamine preparation

Diphenhydramine (**Benadryl**)
or other oral antihistamine
for allergic reactions and itching rashes

Cough medication containing DM *(dextromethorphan)*

Dimenhydrinate (**Gravol**)
suppositories and tablets for nausea and vomiting

Anaesthetic mouth spray such as **Chloraseptic** and lozenges
of any type to soothe a sore throat

Local anaesthetic spray and ointment
for cuts and scrapes such as **Bactine**, or benzocaine (**Solarcaine**)

Antibiotic ointment such as **Polysporin**
for burns and scrapes

Antibiotic eye drops or ear drops such as **Polysporin**
for pink eye and ear infections

Antacid (**Maalox, Riopan, Tums, Rolaids**, etc.)
for heartburn or indigestion

***Check with your pharmacist for advice
about substitutions to this list.***

How to use this book

This self-help book has been designed to assist people, in otherwise good health, to deal with some of life's common health problems. It is not designed to replace your doctor. It was written to give people some of the knowledge needed to better treat these common problems. This book will give you advice that you may receive from a doctor without the inconvenience and expense of an office or emergency room visit.

People with serious medical problems such as severe lung disease, heart disease, kidney failure, diabetes, liver disease, cancer or Aids will frequently need to seek medical assistance earlier to reduce the chance that the chronic or serious medical condition will get worse. If you are unwell and cannot cope you must see your family doctor or go to the hospital.

When we refer to children in this book we mean anyone under 16 years of age.

To use this book properly:

1. Select your topic and read that section thoroughly, from start to finish, before using the advice given.

2. Re-evaluate how you or your child is doing regularly during the illness.

3. Consult your doctor or go to the hospital immediately should you or your child's condition be rapidly changing for the worse. Anyone who appears very ill should see a doctor promptly.

4. Read this book over BEFORE you need it in an urgent situation. **THE INFORMATION PAGES** will help you make decisions about products you may wish to buy from your local pharmacy.

Initially some charts in this book may look difficult. All questions are answered by a "YES" or "NO". Just follow the arrows and you will find it very user friendly.

What do you need?

You must be genuinely interested

Keep this book in a handy place where you can easily find it whenever you have a health problem. Use this book to improve your skills in caring for yourself and your family. It would also be a good idea to take **THIS BOOK** with you when you are travelling or on vacation. Proper and timely use of this book may save you from making unnecessary hospital or doctor visits.

You will need some tools

Making wise decisions about health problems is easier when you have the right tools. **YOU NEED A GOOD THERMOMETER**. Your hand on someone's forehead can give false information. The best thermometer to buy is an electronic digital, with glass thermometers the second best option. Temperature strips are not accurate and should not be trusted. Tympanic or ear thermometers are more difficult to get accurate results from.

If you are using glass thermometers you will need one for oral and one for rectal use. Washing a thermometer in hot water may cause it to break.

See page 5 for more information about taking a temperature.

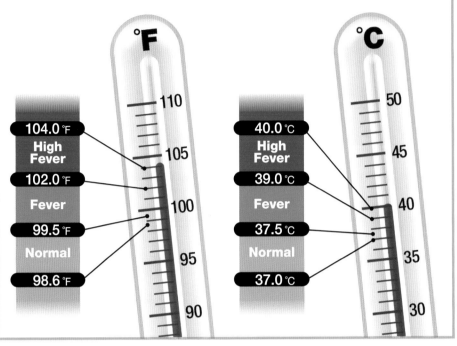

Temperature **ORAL**

°F
- 110
- 105
- 100
- 95
- 90

104.0 °F
High Fever
102.0 °F
Fever
99.5 °F
Normal
98.6 °F

°C
- 50
- 45
- 40
- 35
- 30

40.0 °C
High Fever
39.0 °C
Fever
37.5 °C
Normal
37.0 °C

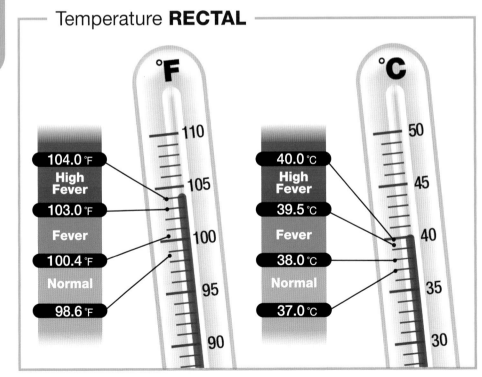

Temperature **RECTAL**

°F
- 110
- 105
- 100
- 95
- 90

104.0 °F
High Fever
103.0 °F
Fever
100.4 °F
Normal
98.6 °F

°C
- 50
- 45
- 40
- 35
- 30

40.0 °C
High Fever
39.5 °C
Fever
38.0 °C
Normal
37.0 °C

 "Did you know that fever may help us fight infections? However, we often feel better if we treat the fever."

Fever
What you should know about fever

A fever, or an elevated body temperature, is usually a symptom of infection and not usually a problem of itself. It is one of the ways that we fight infection. If the fever is not causing a problem, you do not have to treat it, though you will often feel a lot better if the fever is treated. A fever should prompt a parent to watch for a source of infection. Viral infections do not have specific treatments. If the fever is high or prolonged despite home therapy, then a visit to your family doctor is advised. Children under 3 months of age, anyone on chemotherapy, anyone with a serious ongoing disease, and those who have had recent surgery should seek medical advice about all fevers.

What is fever?

	Normal	Fever	High Fever
Temperature Orally (taken by mouth)	up to 37.5°C (99.5°F)	37.5 - 39.0°C 99.5 - 102°F	over 39.0°C over 102°F
Temperature Rectally (taken by rectum)	up to 38.0°C (100.4°F)	38.0 - 39.5°C 100.4 - 103°F	over 39.5°C over 103°F

Keep in mind that body temperature may rise with exercise, with overdressing, after a hot bath, or as a result of very hot weather. Be sure to recheck a temperature you are unsure of in 30 to 60 minutes.

How to take a temperature

When taking a temperature you must have the right equipment. You cannot depend on the feel of a forehead with your hand to determine someone's temperature accurately. As discussed on page 3 we recommend you obtain either an electronic or glass thermometer. Temperatures are best taken rectally or orally. You should take a look at the thermometer before use and note how you have to rotate the glass to see the mercury or alcohol. As noted above, the oral temperature may be lower than the rectal temperature because the mouth is cooled by breathing. Be sure you shake the glass thermometer down below 37°C or 99°F before using it.

AN ORAL TEMPERATURE may be used in older children or adults.
Oral temperatures may be falsely high or low depending on recent hot or cold drinks. Wait about 10 minutes after drinking to take an oral temperature.

A RECTAL TEMPERATURE is more accurate and should be performed if possible. This is important in young children who may not cooperate for an oral temperature or may bite a glass thermometer. *Taking a rectal temperature does not hurt the child.*

How to take a RECTAL temperature

1. Lay the child over your lap.
2. Lubricate the thermometer with **Vaseline** or other lubricant.
3. Hold the thermometer about 1 inch from the end to prevent insertion more than 1 inch. Do not force it.
4. Read the temperature after 2 minutes with a glass thermometer, or when the electronic thermometer "beeps".

We feel that armpit temperatures and skin temperature strips are inaccurate and are not advised.

How to take an ORAL temperature

1. Place the oral thermometer under the tongue on one side or the other towards the back of the mouth.
2. Be certain that it is being held by the lips, not by the teeth.
3. Leave the thermometer in place for 3 minutes before reading the temperature.
4. If the child cannot nose breathe because of congestion, you can suction out the nose first with a small suction bulb. Mouth breathing while taking the temperature will falsely lower the temperature.

5

Topics for Mother and Newborn Child

INTRODUCTION

This section is intended to help new mothers and their families deal with some of the most common health issues that affect them and their newborn babies, the problems that arise shortly after delivery and during the first year of baby's life. Many of these issues are not illnesses but common things that happen to most new mothers and babies, which can cause unnecessary worry and stress. Although most of these common complaints have several possible solutions, often there is no one "perfect" answer. This information will not replace your doctor, but hopefully it will allow you to deal with many issues on your own and help guide you to decide when a doctor visit is needed.

The most important thing to remember is that you will have some discomfort after giving birth, and will also be easily fatigued. This will limit your ability to do everything around the house, but it is more important to look after yourself and your baby. Don't worry about the smaller day-to-day issues. Get your rest and make a little time each day for you. Your baby will only be a baby once so try to relax and enjoy these early months.

How to make the best of your doctor visits

Standard post-delivery care

If you see your family doctor or midwife for care during your pregnancy and delivery, they will continue to care for you and your baby after delivery. If you have seen an obstetrician for the delivery, they will want to see you after the delivery and will refer your baby for care with your family doctor or a pediatrician. Most babies do not need to see a specialist for routine care. Your family doctor will refer you to a pediatrician if necessary.

Mothers are usually seen for a routine post-delivery check-up about 6 weeks after delivery. If there were any complications during late pregnancy or delivery, your doctor may want to see you sooner. During this visit, you should expect an examination including blood pressure, pelvic exam, PAP test and a check of wound repairs. If there were any problems during pregnancy, such as toxemia, diabetes or high blood pressure, these problems will also be reviewed. Blood tests to check blood counts (hemoglobin) might be ordered. You should also have a discussion with your doctor about birth control during this visit, and remember that breast-feeding does not offer effective birth control.

Most doctors will want to see your baby within the first week of birth (5 to 10 days of age). During this visit, they will conduct a general examination, check the baby's weight, assess feeding and answer any pressing questions you have. It is important that you come prepared for this visit—you may feel overwhelmed by the first few days and need to make yourself a short list of the most important issues.

Further appointments for your baby will normally be planned for 1, 2, 4, 6, 9 and 12 months. These appointments are to assess growth and developmental milestones. At these appointments the doctor will repeat the general examination and administer immunizations as required.

If you have any problems between appointments you should contact your doctor to make arrangements for a special appointment.

When you see your doctor

Most women have had several visits with their doctor during their pregnancy so that by the time they deliver their baby, they are comfortable in the relationship. Being able to talk to your doctor and communicate clearly with each other is the single most important factor in your relationship.

Before your appointments it is often helpful to make a short list of the issues that are most important to you and your baby. This can be limitless, but the time your doctor has for you at any one appointment is not. We suggest that you bring up the most important issues first. If you have issues that don't seem to be dealt with to your satisfaction then you should make a special appointment to deal with them separately.

Babies cannot tell you how they are feeling so it can be difficult to know exactly what the problem is. The best way to find the solution to a problem is to see your doctor again if the problem persists. Often a repeat check-up will help you both arrive at a proper diagnosis and solution.

Breast-feeding

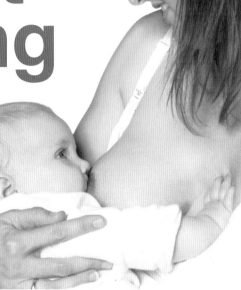

Introduction

Breast milk is human milk for human babies. It is nutritional, convenient and inexpensive. Breast milk may provide protection from infection as it contains antibodies that fight infection, as well as protection from illnesses like asthma and diabetes. Breast-feeding may also protect mothers from developing breast and ovarian cancer.

Even though breast-feeding is natural and possible for almost all mothers and their babies, it is sometimes difficult to get started. The following are some steps, which can lead to successful breast-feeding.

1. Before delivery, learn about breast-feeding. Search out breast-feeding support groups; attend prenatal classes; read books; watch videos.

2. At delivery, have the baby placed on your tummy as soon as possible. Studies have shown that babies instinctively move to and will latch onto the breast in the first hour after birth. This can be a very positive first step to getting the feeding off to a good start.

3. Learn what a good latch is and what effective nursing feels like.

4. Accept support from your husband, family, public health nurses, lactation specialists and interested friends.

How breast milk changes

1. From birth to about day 3 the breasts will produce a thick yellow fluid. This is called colostrum and it is high in vitamins, proteins and antibodies to protect your baby from infection. It is also a mild laxative that helps babies move their bowels.

2. From day 3 to day 10, early milk is produced. It contains more water.

3. From day 10 on, mature milk is produced. This milk is unique in that it changes its make-up during each feed, with the fat content increasing during the feed. This means that most of the fat is passed to baby near the end of the feeding.

4. Breast milk has more fat than protein (60% to 40%), while formula is usually the opposite, 40% fat and 60% protein.

5. Formula is nutritious but it is not the same as breast milk.

The latch

A proper latch makes it easier for the baby to eat and causes fewer problems for mother.

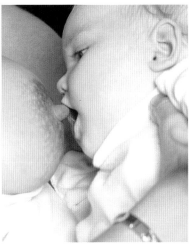

▶ Cradle baby firmly with baby's mouth facing your breast. Support baby's head with one hand, while pressing baby's bottom against your chest.

▶ Wait for baby's mouth to open wide, then pull the baby onto the breast letting the chin hit the breast first. Don't put the breast into baby's mouth. Baby's lips should be flared back on the breast.

▶ The nipple should be in the top of baby's mouth. There should be no pain when baby sucks.

▶ The areola (coloured part of the breast around the nipple) should be covered by and in baby's mouth. It is most important that the lower half of the areola be covered.

▶ While nursing, the baby's chin should be well under the breast and nose very close to the skin of the breast.

▶ If well latched, gentle pulling away should not break the latch. There should be little or no pain felt at the nipple.

▶ Most mothers find that sitting upright with baby in the cradle position is easiest. Try lying down, sitting on a bed or other positions only after breast-feeding is well established.

▶ A pillow on your lap may help support a bigger or heavier baby. This is very helpful if you have had a C-section.

▶ If you don't have a proper latch, take the baby off and try again. Letting the baby feed with a poor latch will cause pain and poor feeding.

▶ If the breast or nipples are painful take the baby off and start again. Don't let the baby "nipple" feed. See **BREAST PAIN** page 46.

▶ Don't worry about anything else—they can wait.

▶ Relax!!! Have a warm drink. Let people help. Accept the support of husband, family, and professionals. It never hurts to hear that you are doing a great job either.

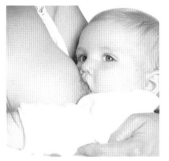

Is baby getting enough breast milk?

Proper suckling

Once baby is latched on, they will suck. This is a specific series of movements:

1. Baby opens mouth wider
2. Baby pauses as milk flows into the mouth
3. Baby closes mouth

These pattern repeats until the mouth is full and the baby swallows. You should be able to see and hear the baby swallow.

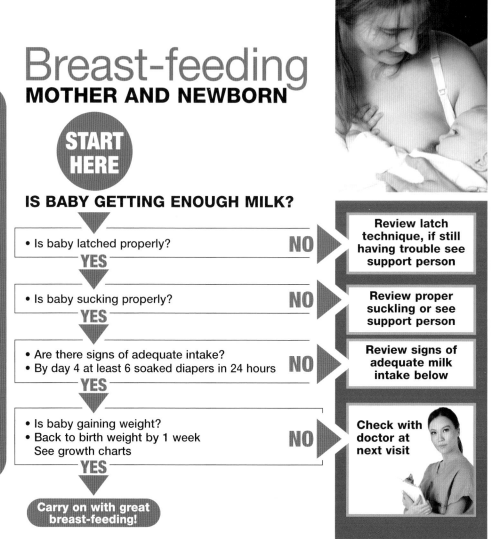

Breast-feeding
MOTHER AND NEWBORN

START HERE

IS BABY GETTING ENOUGH MILK?

- Is baby latched properly? **NO** → Review latch technique, if still having trouble see support person

YES

- Is baby sucking properly? **NO** → Review proper suckling or see support person

YES

- Are there signs of adequate intake?
- By day 4 at least 6 soaked diapers in 24 hours **NO** → Review signs of adequate milk intake below

YES

- Is baby gaining weight?
- Back to birth weight by 1 week
  See growth charts **NO** → Check with doctor at next visit

YES

Carry on with great breast-feeding!

Is baby getting enough milk?

By day 4 or 5, babies who are drinking well will have at least 6 soaked diapers every 24 hours.

Bowel movements change over the first few weeks. From birth to about day 3, the movements are tarry and black. This is called meconium.

After this, movements become seedy and yellow and can be passed 5 to 10 times daily.

After about 3 weeks, the stools become more yellow and soft, then brown as solid food is added. Movements may continue as frequently as after every feeding or may occur only once every 7 to 12 days.

How often should I feed?

From birth to day 3, you should offer the breast approximately every 1 to 3 hours during the day and every 3 to 4 hours at night. Sleepy babies may not be getting enough food, so you have to wake them to feed. Be sure to review "Is baby getting enough milk?"

After day 3, most babies will develop a pattern. Feeding schedules will vary from every 2 to 4 hours during the day and every 3 to 4 hours at night. With time, babies take more milk at every feeding as their stomachs grow and the time between feeds will lengthen. When babies will sleep through the night is quite variable.

Saving milk

Milk can be expressed from the breasts and saved for later use. It is best to express milk after baby has finished a feeding. Milk can be expressed manually by "milking" the breast between both hands or with a pump. We recommend using an electric pump. Rubber bulb pumps are not recommended.

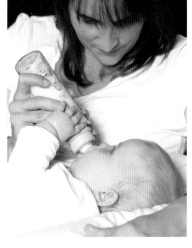

Expressed milk should be stored in a sterile container. Heat glass containers for 15 minutes in the oven at 225°F/110°C. Milk can be stored for up to 5 days if refrigerated. If frozen, milk may be stored as follows:

- Refrigerator freezer for 2 weeks
- Self-contained freezer for 3 to 4 months
- Deep-freeze (0°F, -16°C) for 6 months

It is important not to cook the milk while thawing, so do not use a microwave or place it in boiling water—either let the milk thaw at room temperature or hold the bottle under a warm running tap. The milk will appear to have separated after thawing because the water and fat thaw separately. Just shake the milk gently and it will mix again.

When do I wean my baby?

There is no right answer to this question except that you should wean the baby when you are ready. Many of us have outside pressures that make breast-feeding difficult to continue, so you should not feel guilty if you have to wean your baby. Having accomplished even a few weeks of breast-feeding is terrific. Most experts would suggest that in a perfect world, the only necessary food for a child under the age of 2 years is breast milk.

If you wean your baby before the age of 1 year, you should replace the breast milk with a formula until the baby is at least 9 to 12 months of age. Please see **FORMULA FEEDING** page 13.

Homogenized milk (3% fat) can be use instead of formula after baby is 1 year old. Do not use 2% milk until your child is 2 years old. Avoid 1% or skim milk until they are over 2 years old.

Bottles, soothers and extra fluids

While breast-feeding, you should not need to give your baby any extra fluids. If you want to introduce a bottle so others can feed when you are busy you should do so only after breast-feeding is well established. Breast-feeding is a little more work than bottle-feeding and like most of us your baby will be as lazy as possible. You can feed the baby either formula or stored breast milk in the bottle. You can also try cup feeding older babies.

You should avoid pacifiers or soothers until breast-feeding is going well.

Babies should not require extra water or juice until 12 to 24 months. Avoid sweet juices until children are 2 to 5 years of age.

Other Frequently Asked Questions about Breast-feeding

Do mothers have to eat a special diet while breast-feeding?

No. Mom's diet does not affect breast milk, nor do mothers have to drink milk to make milk. Nursing mothers need to take more calcium to prevent excess loss of calcium from their bones. The simplest source of calcium is cow's milk, so drinking three 8oz glasses per day is recommended for nursing moms. Apart from that, mom's diet should be well-rounded. Occasionally, moms will notice that their baby gets "fussy" after she has eaten a certain food, spice or food prepared in a certain way. Common sense would suggest that mom should avoid that food until baby is weaned.

Should nursing mothers avoid all medications while breast-feeding?

In general, physicians do not like mothers to take medications while they are pregnant because they may affect the baby's growth or the development of the baby's organs. Concerns about medications passing through the breast milk of nursing mothers is not as great, and in fact, many medications will not harm the baby. The best approach is to let your doctor know about any medications you are taking, including herbal products or supplements. On the flip side, you should always let any prescribing doctor know that you are breast-feeding so they can check on the safety of the medication.

Do babies always eat the same amount each day?

No. Babies will go through "growth spurts" every 4 to 6 weeks and mothers may feel that they cannot make enough milk to satisfy their baby. The best approach is to feed the baby on demand. When you increase the frequency of feeding, the breasts will usually respond and "catch up" to the baby's demands in 1 to 2 days. This increased feeding rate will avoid the need to offer supplemental formula or other fluids, and using supplements may prevent the breast from achieving the natural "catch up".

If we sterilize bottles, why don't mothers have to wash their nipples before feeding?

Washing normally with a sponge or cloth during the daily shower is all that is required to keep the nipples healthy. The milk is sterile within the breast. Applying creams, lotions or soap to the nipples frequently may result in a drying of the nipples with painful cracking.

What do I do with sore nipples?

It is more common than not for mother's nipples to become sore following the start of breast-feeding. Nipples usually adapt to feeding within a week or so. You may find that if you rub a little milk over the nipple following the feed and let the breast air dry may help. Sometimes, however, sore nipples are caused by a yeast infection. Check the baby's mouth for white spots that peel off, but do not wash off.

Formula or Bottle-feeding

There are many commercial formulas available which can be used for babies who are not breast-fed until 9 to 12 months of age. If you do feed your baby formula, it should be iron fortified. There are two main types of formula: cow's milk and soy-based. The latter should be used for those babies who either are allergic to or are not able to digest the cow's milk formula well.

Formula comes as a ready-to-eat liquid or as a concentrate, liquid or powder, which is mixed with water. Follow the mixing instructions exactly to provide proper nutrition.

Feeding instructions for age	Age	Frequency of feeds	Volume of each feeding
	1-14 days	2-4 hrs	2-3oz
	2-8 weeks	3-4 hrs	4-5oz
	2-3 months	4-5 hrs	5-6oz
	3-6 months	5-6 hrs	6-8oz
	9-12 months	3 per day	6-8oz

Formula or Bottle-feeding

IS MY FORMULA-FED BABY GETTING ENOUGH TO EAT?

START HERE

Before you start this flowchart, be certain that you have followed the mixing and preparation instructions accurately for the commercial formula that you have purchased.

Check the chart above to determine the frequency and volume of feeds that are appropriate for your child.

- Does baby spit up the majority of feeds after feeding? *or*
- Is the baby forcefully vomiting? *or*
- Are there less than 5 soaked diapers every 24 hours? *or*
- Is there less than 1 bowel movement per day? *or*
- Is there blood in the urine or bowel movement? *or*
- Are the baby's eyes or skin yellow coloured? *or*
- Is there a new rash? *or*
- Is the baby losing weight or not gaining weight?

YES ▶ **See Your Doctor**

NO

Continue with feeding according to the chart

Feeding beyond Breast or Bottle

When should you introduce solid food to your new baby? Just when things seem to be going well with respect to breast or bottle-feeding, many parents become concerned that they should be moving on to solid food. Often friends and family will give advice based on baby's sleeping habits, size or mood, but generally there is no need to give a baby anything other than breast milk or formula until at least 4 months and often 6 months of age. Giving solids prior to 4 months of age does not help babies sleep through the night as long as they are receiving adequate breast milk or formula.

Babies under 1 year of age get very little nutrition from solid food and depend on breast milk or formula as their main source of energy and nutrition. In fact, it may well be unhealthy to introduce solids too soon. Food allergies are rare, but as a general rule, new solid foods should be introduced one at a time and no more than one new food every 5 to 7 days. This time frame gives you an opportunity to see if there is a problem with the new food. New foods should only be given once a day to start, often quite dilute and in small amounts (1 to 2 tsp), using a small spoon. Timing baby's meals with family meal times is practical and good training.

Feeding Baby Solids

 START HERE *When your baby is 4 to 6 months old and can hold their head up well*

TRY 1 TO 2 TEASPOONS OF DILUTE RICE CEREAL

• Baby moves the food to the back of mouth and baby will swallow well, and there are no problems with vomiting or bowels

NO → **Delay further trials of solids for one week**

YES

May introduce new foods in a similar way, new food every 5 to 7 days in 1 to 2 teaspoons to start

Which foods in what order?

1. Vegetables by 7 months. You can use commercially prepared or freshly cooked and strained. You should try yellow and orange before green vegetables.

2. Fruits should only be introduced after vegetables are well established.

3. Meats are often introduced by 9 months, with white meats (chicken, turkey) first.

4. Eggs/dairy should be introduced between 9 and 12 months.

Finger foods like low salt/sugar crackers or cereals can be given by 9 months. Avoid puddings, desserts and juices until after 2 years of age.

Jaundice

In the first week of life, many healthy, full-term babies and most premature babies will develop jaundice, most commonly on the second or third day of life. You should not be alarmed, as some experts would call this "normal."

Jaundice causes a yellowing of the skin and the eyes. It is not a disease, and usually occurs because your baby's liver isn't mature enough to break down a substance called bilirubin. Unless the levels of bilirubin get unusually high, jaundice will not cause your baby harm, and most jaundice needs no treatment.

Breast-feeding can increase the chances of jaundice, but the overall benefits of breast-feeding far outweigh the risks involved. Prematurity and a lot of bruising during birth can also increase the chances of jaundice.

MY BABY IS YELLOW (JAUNDICED)

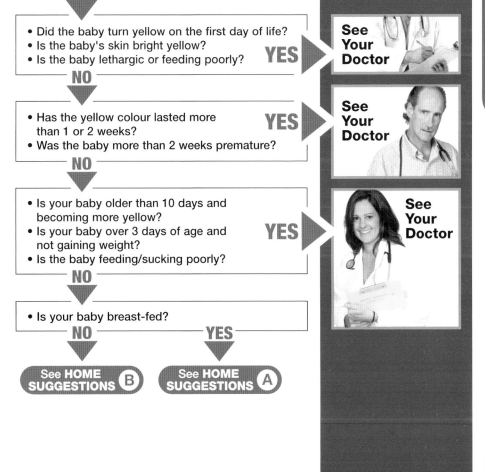

- Did the baby turn yellow on the first day of life?
- Is the baby's skin bright yellow?
- Is the baby lethargic or feeding poorly?

YES → **See Your Doctor**

NO

- Has the yellow colour lasted more than 1 or 2 weeks?
- Was the baby more than 2 weeks premature?

YES → **See Your Doctor**

NO

- Is your baby older than 10 days and becoming more yellow?
- Is your baby over 3 days of age and not gaining weight?
- Is the baby feeding/sucking poorly?

YES → **See Your Doctor**

NO

- Is your baby breast-fed?

NO → See **HOME SUGGESTIONS** B

YES → See **HOME SUGGESTIONS** A

Breast-feeding and Jaundice

▶HOME SUGGESTIONS

HOME SUGGESTIONS Ⓐ

Jaundice is more common in breast-fed babies. This is usually because breast-fed babies may take a few days to develop a good latch and suck. In addition, breast milk production may take a few days increase to meet the baby's needs. Feeding more frequently will stimulate the breasts to produce more milk. The extra feedings may also cause more frequent bowel movements in the baby. These two factors help keep the bilirubin level down.

If you find breast-feeding difficult, you should seek help from a lactation specialist. **Do not quit breast-feeding!** Mother's milk is the best food for your baby. Jaundice may last a little longer in a breast-fed baby than one that is formula-fed, but this is not a serious issue. Please read **HOME SUGGESTIONS** Ⓑ.

HOME SUGGESTIONS Ⓑ

While sunlight does help treat the jaundice, we do not recommend that you undress your baby and put them in the sunlight. To be effective, the ultra violet light must be on the whole body and your baby is very likely to get cold. Direct sunlight can burn a baby's skin very easily.

Feed your baby more frequently. Doing this causes your baby to have more frequent bowel movements and there is less chance to absorb bilirubin from the bowel.

Umbilical Cord Care

SUMMARY: Immediately after birth the umbilical cord is clamped and cut. The small amount of the cord that remains attached to the baby will gradually dry up and then fall off leaving the belly button, usually 3 to 7 days after birth. There is little care required other than keeping the cord area clean and dry with warm water and mild soap. Wiping with alcohol should be avoided because this can increase the chance of infection. If there are signs of infection you should see the doctor.

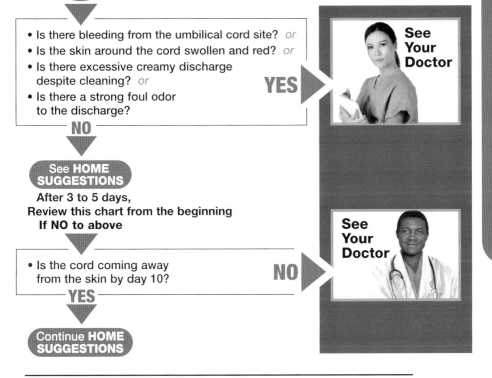

START HERE

- Is there bleeding from the umbilical cord site? *or*
- Is the skin around the cord swollen and red? *or*
- Is there excessive creamy discharge despite cleaning? *or*
- Is there a strong foul odor to the discharge?

YES → See Your Doctor

NO

See **HOME SUGGESTIONS**

After 3 to 5 days,
Review this chart from the beginning
If NO to above

- Is the cord coming away from the skin by day 10?

NO → See Your Doctor

YES

Continue **HOME SUGGESTIONS**

►HOME SUGGESTIONS

1   Keep the cord clean and dry. Use warm water and mild soap to cleanse the area with every diaper change. Do not use alcohol unless instructed by your doctor.

2   Keep the cord away from the top of baby's diaper. Excessive rubbing may pull the cord away too early and cause bleeding.

3   Do not cover the cord with the diaper. Leaving the cord exposed to the air will allow it to keep dry.

4   A small amount of liquid discharge is normal. This usually arises from the base of the cord. It should clear away easily with simple cleaning and not accumulate to any significant amount between cleaning times.

Diaper Rash

SUMMARY: Diaper rash is the most common infant rash. It is usually not serious but can be very uncomfortable for the baby. The rash is usually bright red, can be almost like scalded skin and is confined to skin under the diaper. It is caused by a chemical irritation of the skin due to contact with urine and stool. Frequent changing and allowing the skin to be exposed to air help prevent diaper rash. Sometimes the rash becomes infected with yeast (candida). The hallmarks of this type of infection are the so-called satellite lesions, which are small red spots away from the main rash area. Usually the skin creases (i.e. at the top of the legs) are spared of diaper rash but may become infected in a yeast infection. Although yeast infections may require a prescription medication from your doctor, they frequently respond to a home remedy available without a prescription. If diaper rash does not improve after 3 to 4 days of therapy you should see your doctor.

START HERE

THERE IS A RED, WELL-DEFINED RASH UNDER THE DIAPER AREA

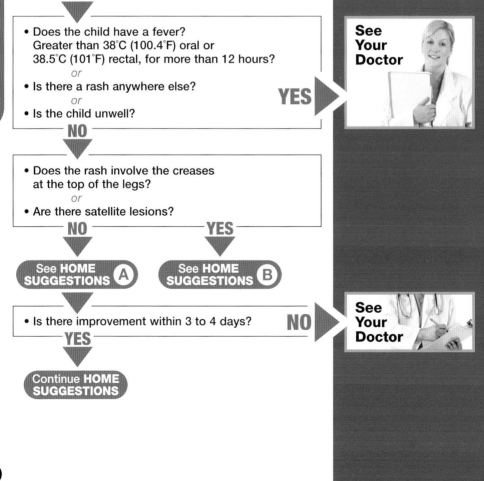

- Does the child have a fever?
  Greater than 38°C (100.4°F) oral or
  38.5°C (101°F) rectal, for more than 12 hours?
  or
- Is there a rash anywhere else?
  or
- Is the child unwell?

YES → **See Your Doctor**

NO

- Does the rash involve the creases at the top of the legs?
  or
- Are there satellite lesions?

NO — See **HOME SUGGESTIONS** Ⓐ

YES — See **HOME SUGGESTIONS** Ⓑ

- Is there improvement within 3 to 4 days? **NO** → **See Your Doctor**

YES

Continue **HOME SUGGESTIONS**

Diaper Rash

▶ HOME SUGGESTIONS

HOME SUGGESTIONS Ⓐ

1 Diaper rash is due to contact of the skin with urine or stool. Letting the baby "air out" with a plastic cover on the bed or floor can be very helpful. Frequent diaper changes are important to reduce the amount of time the skin is in contact with the urine or stool.

2 Barrier creams (**Zincofax**, **Vaseline**, **Peniten** or any zinc oxide cream) are very helpful in reducing the exposure of the skin to urine or stool. They should be applied as a thick layer and not rubbed in.

3 Diet does not usually cause diaper rash, but some babies do seem to get a rash with certain foods. If this is the case with your baby you should avoid the culprit food.

4 Some babies are sensitive to commercial baby wipes, disposable diapers or laundry soaps. These may cause an irritant rash, which is different from true diaper rash. Warm water and mild soap is best for cleaning the diaper area. Avoid products that clearly irritate the skin.

HOME SUGGESTIONS Ⓑ

See 1 to 4 above

Section B refers specifically to diaper rash complicated by yeast.

Often medication is required to clear up a yeast infection. You can try a combination of 0.5% hydrocortisone cream mixed with clotrimazole topical cream in a 50:50 mixture. This should be applied in a thin film to the affected area and rubbed in well about 4 times daily then cover with a barrier cream as outlined in step 2 above. Both of these creams are available without a prescription. Ask your pharmacist for help.

If there is no improvement after 3 to 4 days or if the rash is getting worse despite treatment you should see your doctor.

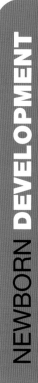

NEWBORN **DEVELOPMENT**

Crying

SUMMARY: All babies cry. It is their only way of making needs known and it is the beginning of verbalization. Most times crying is due to a need or discomfort and settles once that need is satisfied. Many infants seem to have "fussy times" where crying spells are particularly loud and long, which are sometimes attributed to colic. While we do not really know what causes colic, some speculate that it is caused by intestinal pain or cramps. Typically, the baby has a firm or distended belly and draws their legs up. Some will clench their fists and they may become very red in the face. Occasionally passing gas or stool seems to give relief. Rocking, walking, keeping baby upright or holding them like a football over the forearm may all help. Fortunately, most often babies just seem to need to get through this phase and will outgrow these episodes by age 12 to 16 weeks. We believe there is no such thing as spoiling a baby by holding and cuddling them when they are distressed. However, once a parent is sure their baby is safe, well, warm, dry and not hungry, letting the infant cry for 15 to 20 minutes will often allow you to get some needed sleep and will not cause the baby any harm.

MY BABY IS CRYING

- Is the baby ill?
  (Fever, not eating, more irritable than usual)
- Is the baby wet or soiled?
- Is the baby hungry?
- Is the baby hot or cold?
- Is there any danger?

YES

Care for the specific need, then allow the infant to settle

NO

- Let baby attempt to settle for 10 to 15 minutes

Baby does not settle - Consider Colic

See **HOME SUGGESTIONS**

Crying

Suggestions for colic

1 There are no absolute answers. Most babies outgrow colic by 3 months of age.

2 If new foods have recently been introduced, it may be advisable not to give that food to the baby again for 1 or 2 weeks. This is rarely the cause of the problem but there is little harm in holding back some food items for a short period of time.

3 Holding the baby upright and attempting to burp the baby may help. Some parents find the "football" hold helpful while walking with the baby and patting their back. Sometimes getting into the car and going for a drive may help.

4 None of the over-the-counter colic medications have been shown to be of any use. They are not harmful but may be expensive.

5 Mother's diet (while breast-feeding) does not cause colic; however, if a baby is always fussy after mom has a certain meal then avoiding that food won't hurt.

6 If the infant has a possible discomfort such as teething or earache, using acetaminophen (**Tylenol** and others) or ibuprofen (**Advil**, **Motrin** and others) is a good idea. However, avoid medication if there is not an obvious source of discomfort. As colic tends to be a daily (often almost by the clock) occurrence, using pain medication is not a good idea. It rarely helps.

7 Some experts believe that colic is more common in very active infants and that over stimulation may play a role in causing it. A quiet, soothing environment may be helpful. Soothers or pacifiers may also be helpful.

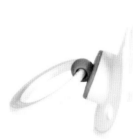
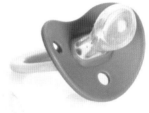

Runny Eyes

SUMMARY: Many new parents are concerned when their child has runny eyes. The most common reason for runny, but otherwise normal eyes, is a blocked tear duct. This is the tube that drains the tears from the eyes to the nose. This discharge is occasionally thicker and can become discoloured. This thicker discharge may be a sign of infection. Sometimes irritants such as smoke or chemicals in creams or powders can cause the eyes to become red. An allergy, which may also be a cause of red eyes in older children or adults, is quite uncommon in babies less than 1 year of age. Occasionally a baby may poke themselves in the eye, and if they scratch the eye, it may become red and runny. Minor infections do not usually cause obvious pain. If the child has painful eyes the doctor should see them.

Eye infections in babies less than 3 months of age are more serious than infections in older babies, and you should see your doctor. Eye infections are very contagious and caregivers must be very careful about handwashing before and after caring for baby's eyes.

START HERE

See the flowchart to help decide the best way to help your child with runny eyes.

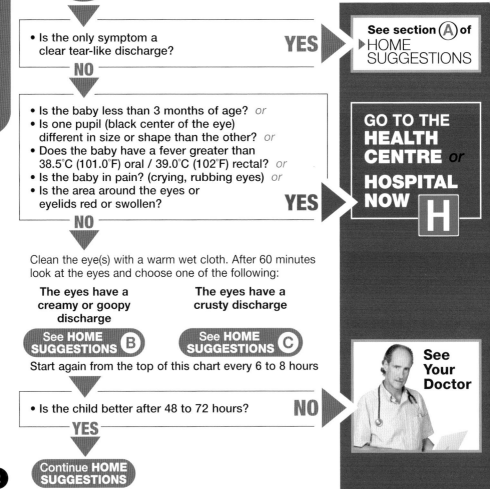

• Is the only symptom a clear tear-like discharge?

YES ▶ See section (A) of ▶ HOME SUGGESTIONS

NO

• Is the baby less than 3 months of age? *or*
• Is one pupil (black center of the eye) different in size or shape than the other? *or*
• Does the baby have a fever greater than 38.5°C (101.0°F) oral / 39.0°C (102°F) rectal? *or*
• Is the baby in pain? (crying, rubbing eyes) *or*
• Is the area around the eyes or eyelids red or swollen?

YES ▶ **GO TO THE HEALTH CENTRE *or* HOSPITAL NOW** [H]

NO

Clean the eye(s) with a warm wet cloth. After 60 minutes look at the eyes and choose one of the following:

The eyes have a creamy or goopy discharge

See **HOME SUGGESTIONS** (B)

The eyes have a crusty discharge

See **HOME SUGGESTIONS** (C)

Start again from the top of this chart every 6 to 8 hours

• Is the child better after 48 to 72 hours?

NO ▶ **See Your Doctor**

YES

Continue **HOME SUGGESTIONS**

Runny Eyes

▶ HOME SUGGESTIONS

Ⓐ This is probably a blocked tear duct

1 Massaging the tear ducts will help open them and allow the eye to drain properly. This massaging may be done with each diaper change (about every 2 to 3 hours). The tear duct is located under the lower lid beside the baby's nose. Massage it by applying mild pressure and "milking" the duct up and over the ridge of the bone under the eye. You may see a small amount of material at the small opening of the duct.

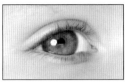

2 Clean the eye and lids with a warm wet cloth as needed.

3 Prevent smoke and other irritants from contacting the baby's eyes.

Ⓑ Goopy eyes For eyes that may have a bacterial infection
(for babies older than 3 months of age)

1 Give 2 drops of a non-prescription antibiotic such as **Polysporin** 4 to 6 times daily. This can be continued for 7 days. If there is no improvement after 2 days of therapy you should see your doctor.

2 Place the drops in the eye by pulling down on the lower lid and placing a drop on the white of the eye; do not drop them directly onto the coloured part of the eye. If your baby keeps their eyes closed, put your baby's face up and place a drop onto the inside corner of the eye. Drops placed here will tend to ooze onto the eye as the baby opens and closes the eyes.

3 You should also place 2 drops 3 to 4 times daily into the unaffected eye. This will reduce the spread of infection.

4 Clean the eye with a warm wet cloth as needed.

5 Warm or cool cloths applied to the eye for 10 minutes each hour may soothe the eyes.

6 Avoid irritants, such as smoke, powders or creams, that will aggravate sore eyes.

Ⓒ Crusty eyes For eyes that may have a viral infection

1 Clean the eyes with warm wet cloths as needed.

2 Warm or cool cloths applied to the eye for 10 minutes each hour may soothe the eyes.

3 Avoid irritants, especially smoke, powders or creams, that may aggravate red or sore eyes.

4 Be very careful about handwashing after caring for baby's eyes because these infections are very contagious.

5 Non-prescription drops for "red eyes" are not recommended for babies.

Runny Nose

SUMMARY: Many babies will have a runny nose from time to time. Because they have smallish nostrils, they seem to get blocked easily. A clear liquid discharge is often due to a viral infection, like the common cold. Thicker coloured discharge may also be caused by a viral infection but occasionally may suggest a bacterial infection for which antibiotics might be helpful. Any baby under 1 year of age with a temperature above 38.5°C or 101°F should be checked by your doctor urgently.

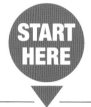

START HERE

- Temperature greater then 38.5°C (101°F) oral / 39°C (102°F) rectal?
  or
- Not eating?
  or
- Not easily awakened?
  or
- Much more irritable?

YES → **GO TO THE HEALTH CENTRE *or* HOSPITAL NOW** **H**

NO

See **HOME SUGGESTIONS**

to treat either clear liquid or coloured discharge

- Have the symptoms improved over 24 to 48 hours?

NO → **See Your Doctor**

YES

Continue **HOME SUGGESTIONS**

Runny Nose

1. Babies have very small nostrils and cannot blow their noses well so need help to clear the secretions. Babies younger than 3 months cannot breathe through their mouths. Because they can only breathe through their nose, a blocked nose is a serious problem that will make feeding difficult and uncomfortable for baby.

2. Liquid discharge can be sucked out using a bulb aspirator which is available at most pharmacies. Gentle suction at the opening of the nose will remove fluid and make breathing easier.

3. Thicker discharge from the nose might be difficult to aspirate with the bulb. Salt water drops (**Salinex** and others) that can be placed (1 to 2 drops) or sprayed as a mist into the nostrils will often loosen up the discharge and make it easier to aspirate.

4. A warm humid environment is best to loosen secretions and let them run out of the nose. A warm air humidifier may be helpful in the baby's room.

5. Warm drinks help to loosen secretions and help them flow from the nose. You may find it easier to clear the nose after feeding.

6. There are decongestants for babies which have variable results, but may be helpful for 1 to 3 days, especially if baby has a bad cold. We prefer baby **Triaminic** drops.

7. If baby has a **FEVER** or **COUGH** see pages 5 and 26 for more information.

NEWBORN DEVELOPMENT

Cough

SUMMARY: Coughing is very common for babies. Occasional coughing is a natural reflex to prevent liquids such as saliva or mucus from entering the lungs. A cough that persists, however, is often a sign of a problem with the baby's airway. This may be due to an abnormally developed airway, a foreign body in the airway or an infection. The problem could lie anywhere in the airway from the nose to the throat, the upper airway tubes, and even into the lungs. The type of cough often makes it possible to know what part of the airway is affected and hence what may be wrong. Nose problems are discussed on page 24. The most common upper airway problem is a viral infection called croup. Common lower airway problems include bronchitis, pneumonia and asthma. Any baby with a persistent cough or a cough associated with troubled breathing should be seen by a physician.

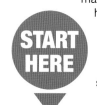

START HERE

- Is your baby having trouble breathing ?
  (see Trouble Breathing on page 27)
  or
- Is baby choking or having trouble swallowing?
  (see Trouble Swallowing on page 27)
  or
- Temperature greater then
  38.5°C (101°F) oral / 39°C (102°F) rectal?
  or
- Does your child look very ill?

YES → **GO TO THE HEALTH CENTRE** *or* **HOSPITAL NOW** **H**

NO / **NO**

Is the cough like a bark or does it sound like a seal?

Probably upper airway problem like croup

Does the cough sound "rattling" as if arising deeper in the chest?

Probably lower airway problem like bronchitis

See **HOME SUGGESTIONS** **A**

See **HOME SUGGESTIONS** **B**

Improving?

Improving?

NO → Persistent cough? Breathing trouble? Swallowing trouble? Continued fever?

YES / **YES**

Continue **HOME SUGGESTIONS** **A**

See **HOME SUGGESTIONS** **B**

See Your Doctor

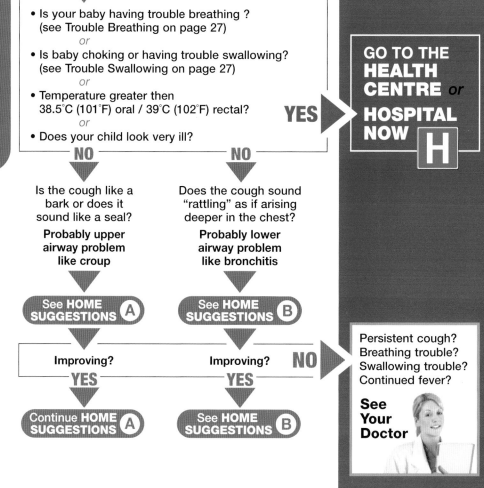

Cough

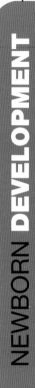
▶ HOME SUGGESTIONS

Trouble breathing

- rapid breathing, more than 60 breaths per minute
- sucking in of skin around neck
- sucking in of ribs
- blue colour of lips, hands or feet

Trouble swallowing

- unable to swallow solids or liquids without choking
- persistent drooling

HOME SUGGESTIONS (A)

1 For mild temperature and discomfort give pain medication such as acetaminophen (**Tylenol** and others) or ibuprofen (**Advil**, **Motrin** and others). See pages 5 and 58.

2 If baby has a **RUNNY NOSE** as well see page 24.

3 A cool mist humidifier may help decrease the swelling of the upper airway that causes the irritation resulting in a croupy cough. Exposure to night air or the mist of a cool shower may bring relief in 10 to 15 minutes. This can be repeated as necessary. If you are unsuccessful in reducing symptoms there is specific drug therapy available at hospital.

4 Avoid cigarette smoke and other environmental irritants.

5 Continue bottle and breast-feeding. More frequent but smaller quantity feeds may be better tolerated.

HOME SUGGESTIONS (B)

1 For mild temperature and discomfort give pain medication such as acetaminophen (**Tylenol** and others) or ibuprofen (**Advil**, **Motrin** and others). See pages 5 and 58.

2 For associated **RUNNY NOSE** see page 24.

3 Continue to breast or bottle-feed as usual. You may have to try smaller feeds more often. Your baby may tire more easily when ill.

4 Avoid cigarette smoke and other irritants.

5 Cough medicine is generally reserved for children over 1 year of age.

Skin Conditions

Changes of the skin are common and result in many doctor visits.
The following section discusses many of the most common skin conditions.

1   Newborns - These are temporary skin changes affecting newborn babies which will go away with time. **No treatment is needed**.

i)   **Milia** • Not to be confused with Monilia. These are white bumps on the face scattered over the nose, cheeks and forehead, about 1mm in size. These are little cysts that occur in about 40% of newborns.

ii)   **Acne** • Very common and appears like acne of adolescence. This appears at about age 3 weeks, usually on the face. This is thought to be more common in breast-fed infants. It will resolve in 6 to 12 months.

iii)   **Sebaceous gland hyperplasia** • These are flat, yellow patches or bumps seen mostly over the nose. These are overgrown sebaceous or sweat glands.

iv)   **Harlequin skin change** • If newborns are on their side, they will sometimes become flushed or red over the whole side of the body they are lying on. This may often be quite obvious as a change down the midline of the body. It will resolve within 20 minutes if the baby's position is changed.

v)   **Mottling** • Cold environments may cause a lace-like pattern of reddish or bluish lines (blood vessels) over the infant's body. This goes away with warming the baby.

vi)   **Erythema toxicum** • This rash occurs in about 50% of babies and is often confused by the parents as an infection. Red patches appear on the body and may develop into yellowish bumps or even small blisters. They usually appear at about 2 days of age and disappear within a week.

vii)   **Miliaria** • Tiny little closely grouped bumps or blisters with or without red skin as a base. These are due to blocked sweat glands usually due to overheating. They go away in a cooler environment.

COMMON SKIN INFECTIONS

2   **Cradle cap** • This white or yellow-red scaly rash looks greasy and involves the scalp and face. It often will settle with daily washing with baby shampoo and a mild "scrub". If it continues see your doctor.

3   **Impetigo** • Open skin that becomes crusted and weeps suggests a bacterial infection. This requires antibiotics. See your doctor.

4   **Diaper rash** • Diaper rash is red sore skin in the diaper area often due to chemical irritation from contact with urine or stool under the warm diaper. Letting the baby's skin "air out" and applying a barrier cream (**Zincofax**, **Peniten** and others) when wearing a diaper will clear this up. These rashes may become infected with yeast (candida). Again, airing out helps. Specific treatment using an antifungal cream (**Conestin**) mixed with a mild steroid cream (Cortate 0.5%) will be very effective. If the rash persists despite treatment for 3 to 5 days you should see your doctor. Also see section entitled **DIAPER RASH** on page 18.

Many viral infections may cause a rash. If you baby is ill with any skin changes you should see your doctor.

Skin Conditions

Cradle cap **Impetigo** **Diaper Rash**

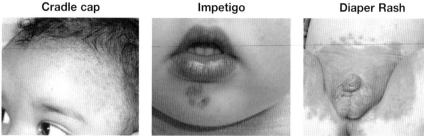

A Word About

Sleeping

Infants have a very different sleep pattern than older children and adults. Normal babies sleep 14 to 16 hours per day, with 9 to 10 hours concentrated sleep at night. About 70% of babies sleep 6 to 8 hours by 6 months of age. Some babies have their days and nights reversed, and only time will fix this problem. Infant sleep cycles are shorter than those of adults, so frequent waking is normal. It is a good idea to allow a baby over the age of 6 months about 15 minutes to resettle themselves if they wake up through the night. Younger infants will often require 1 to 3 feedings through the night.

Circumcision

Many parents find it difficult to know whether or not they should have their male infant circumcised. The bottom line is that this is only about choice. Occasionally there is a medical reason for circumcision but this is rare. On the other hand, there may be reasons to refuse to perform circumcision (i.e. abnormal development of the penis requiring the foreskin be used for reconstruction). For the normal male infant there is no compelling medical reason to be circumcised. Complications include bleeding and infection, which can be serious. Most doctors who perform circumcisions use local anaesthetics so that the baby does not feel pain during the procedure and will tolerate the operation well.

Teething

The appearance of teeth can be a very difficult time for some infants and can occur without warning. Generally the first tooth will erupt at 5 to 6 months of age. The lower middle teeth are usually first and often come in pairs. The upper middle teeth will be next between 6 and 8 months of age. The lower then upper outer front teeth come next between 7 and 11 months. The molars generally don't appear until after baby is 1 year of age. A baby usually has all 20 primary teeth by 30 months. Although these dates are average, many babies will have teeth erupt on entirely different schedules and in different orders.

There are many myths about teething. Some babies increase chewing behaviour or decrease eating while teething, as it can be uncomfortable. Babies do not get a fever because they are teething. Babies are not "ill" because they are teething. A tooth may erupt and then "go back in" or take several days to "break through" the gums. There may be a small amount of bleeding from the gums as the tooth erupts. Allowing the baby to chew often helps. If there is obvious pain (baby is crying) with chewing you can give some pain medication for 2 to 3 days which may help. See page 58 for information about pain medication. Applying products directly onto the gums has not generally been found to be helpful. Rubbing the gums with your finger, however, may be soothing and give some relief. Try it. Your baby will let you know.

Bowel Movements

All newborns should have bowel movements daily for the first week or so. The type of feeding (breast vs. bottle) does not affect the bowel frequency during the first week. The initial stools called meconium, are tarry black and represent a cleaning out of the bowel as it begins to work. Breast-fed babies develop a yellowish seedy looking stool after the first 3 days or so. They continue to have at least one stool per day until they are 7 to 10 days of age. After that, some breast-fed infants will have a bowel movement after every feeding and others will have a bowel movement only once every 10 days or more. As long as the movements remain soft this is not constipation. See page 81 to review **CONSTIPATION**. Infrequent bowel movements indicate excellent absorption of breast milk.

Bottle-fed infants often have soft mushy green or brown stools. Again they should have at least one movement per day after the first week to 10 days, and it is less likely that a bottle-fed baby will go more than 1 or 2 days without a bowel movement.

With the introduction of solids, stools will become more formed, and can be almost any colour of green, brown or yellow-orange, depending on diet. Colour really has no diagnostic significance.

Some babies will pass a small amount of blood with their bowel movements. This may come from the mother's breast if breast-fed. Small cracks in the anal canal, called fissures, can also bleed a small amount. If you see blood in your baby's stools, you should see your doctor, though this is not urgent and a visit within 3 or 5 days as long as everything is going well is acceptable. A visit to the emergency is indicated if your baby is obviously bleeding from the rectal area.

Immunization

A vaccine is a drug which is given to stimulate the formation of antibodies against diseases and thus make the vaccinated person immune to catching the disease if they are exposed to it.

Immunizations are given to children at a very young age. There are many myths about immunization and some parents are concerned about having their children immunized. This chapter contains information to help answer these concerns; however, you should discuss immunization with your own doctor before vaccinating your child.

Immunization is safe and the only absolute reason not to give a vaccination is if your child has an allergy to the vaccine. Immunization is effective in preventing many diseases that can cause serious illness and even death, and over the last few decades, these once common illnesses are almost unheard of due to the vaccination programs. Even those few people who are not vaccinated benefit from vaccination programs by reducing the number of people who can carry an illness and transmit it to the non-immune.

Immunization against diphtheria, polio, tetanus, pertussis (whooping cough), hemophyllis influenza, measles, mumps and rubella are recommended for all children. There are also vaccines for Hepatitis A and B, chicken pox and other infections that be caught when travelling to different areas of the world.

Some children will suffer minor side-effects after vaccination which are easily managed at home. See **HOME SUGGESTIONS** page 33. Serious side-effects are very rare and occur in as few as 1 in one million vaccinations.

Immunizations do not have to be delayed if your child has a minor illness like a cold. Vaccines do not weaken the immune system.

There are no alternatives to vaccination to prevent the common diseases listed below. Vaccination is not mandatory by law, but children who have not been immunized may not be allowed to attend school if there is an outbreak of an illness.

Standard Immunization Schedule

2 months of age	Diphtheria, Polio, Tetanus, Pertussis, Hemophilus Influenza
4 months of age	Diphtheria, Polio, Tetanus, Pertussis, Hemophilus Influenza
6 months of age	Diphtheria, Polio, Tetanus, Pertussis, Hemophilus Influenza
12-15 months of age	Measles, Mumps, Rubella
18 months of age	Diphtheria, Polio, Tetanus, Pertussis, Hemophilus Influenza
4-6 years of age	Diphtheria, Polio, Tetanus, Pertussis, Measles, Mumps, Rubella

Immunization

START HERE

20 minutes to 1 hour before vaccination the child should be given an oral dose of acetaminophen. See page 58 for appropriate dose for weight.

AFTER VACCINATION

- Is there fever over 40.5°C (105°F) rectal or oral?
  or
- Has the child had a fit or seizure within 48 hours of vaccination?
  or
- Has your child developed inconsolable crying within 48 hours of vaccination?
  or
- Has your child become non-responsive and floppy within 48 hours of vaccination?
  or
- Does your child appear to be very ill?

YES ▶ **GO TO THE HEALTH CENTRE** *or* **HOSPITAL NOW** [H]

NO

- Fever over 38.5°C (101°F) rectal / 38°C (100.4°F) oral?
  or
- Is the injection site very red and swollen?
  or
- Is the baby very fussy?

YES ▶ **See next page** ▶HOME SUGGESTIONS

NO

Review every 6 hours for 2 days.

- Have the symptoms resolved within 2 days?   **NO** ▶ **See Your Doctor**

YES

Continue Routine Vaccination Schedule

NEWBORN DEVELOPMENT

Immunization

▶ HOME SUGGESTIONS

1   Many infants have pain at the site of the injection. Some will develop redness, swelling or a lump. This can be treated with cold compresses—using ice wrapped in a damp cloth or just a cold damp cloth for about five minutes every hour while baby is awake may help. Most local reactions resolve over a few days, though sometimes there will be small lump that persists which you should show to your doctor. Acetaminophen (**Tylenol** and others) will help with any pain. We do not recommend the use of other pain or fever medications following vaccinations.

2   Low-grade fever is common after vaccination. Acetaminophen (**Tylenol** and others) every 4 to 6 hours is helpful. We do not recommend other pain or fever medications following vaccination. The fever should go away in 1 or 2 days, but if it persists, see your doctor.

3   A mild illness with runny nose, mild fever and a red rash on the face and body is occasionally seen 7 to 10 days after immunization for measles, mumps and rubella.

4   Soothe your baby being careful to avoid contact with the injection site.

5   More than 99% of infants have no reaction to their immunization and many don't even react at the time of their needle.

6   You should inform your doctor if your baby has had any reaction to eating eggs (i.e. around 1 year of age). This was thought to be a reason not to vaccinate with MMR (measles, mumps and rubella) but this is no longer the case.

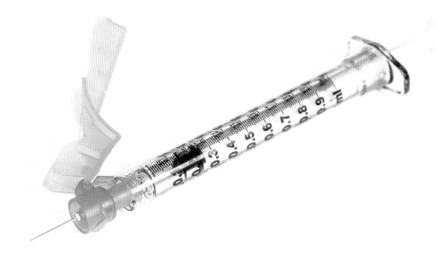

Development

Babies tend to follow a pattern know as "milestones" of development for physical activities (motor skills), language and thinking. A baby who does not achieve these "milestones" may be showing signs of illness or developmental delay. Well baby exams with your doctor are in part a check of the baby's development. The table reproduced in this section is only a guide to normal "milestones" and is included for parental interest only—it is not intended for diagnosing development delay. If you have concerns about your baby's development, you should speak to your doctor at the next scheduled appointment. Babies do best when they have lots of contact with parents and siblings: you should talk frequently to your baby, using normal language. It is also never too early to begin sharing books with your baby. Infants thrive on lots of interaction and activities—TV, radio and other sources of voice are no substitute for loving human contact and stimulation.

Milestones of Development

Time	Gross Motor	Fine Motor	Communication	Thinking
first month	• lies with arms/legs flexed, turns head	nil	• may fixate on face prefers human face	?
after 1 month	• can hold head briefly in line with body • arms and legs extend more	nil	• starts to follow objects i.e. faces sound	?
by 8 weeks	• holds head steady while sitting	nil	• smiles to face and voice • starts to "coo" with familiar people	• will stare at spot an object disappears from
by 4 months	• no head lag when pulled from lying to sitting • brings hands together in midline	• grasps rattle • reaches • transfers between hands	• will listen to music • says ahh, nahh, laughs	• excited by food • cries when parents leave • stares at own hand
by 6 months	• sits without support • rolls back to front		• babbles in single syllables	
by 8 months	• supports weight • likes to bounce	• uses thumb and finger to grasp	• starts to "no" • will do 1 step communication with gestures	• uncovers hidden objects • bangs blocks together
by 10 months	• "cruises" around furniture		• step 1 communication with voice "mama, dada" • waves bye-bye	• plays peek-a-boo • responds to name
1 year	• walks	• turns pages	• first real word	• does pretend play

Growth

Infants tend to grow at a predictable rate. While there is a wide variety in babies' height and weight, once they begin to grow they tend to do so following a given "percentile" of normal. For example, a baby who is at the 60th percentile for height and weight is taller and heavier than 59% of babies their age, and shorter and lighter than 39% of babies of the same age, and will grow at the same percentile give or take 10 to 15%. Your doctor will follow your baby's growth as an indication of health. We have included a typical growth chart for your interest and to record your baby's growth.

Birth to 36 months: Boys
Length-for-age and Weight-for-age percentiles

NAME _____

RECORD # _____

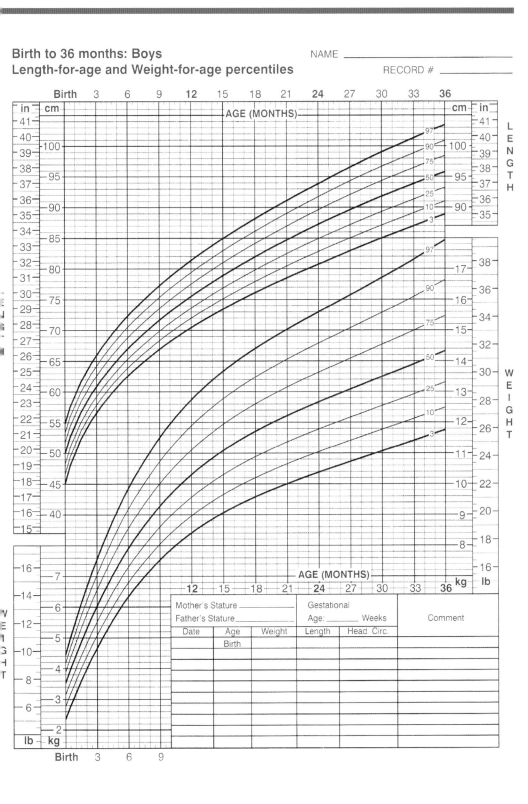

Birth to 36 months: Girls
Length-for-age and Weight-for-age percentiles

NAME _____

RECORD # _____

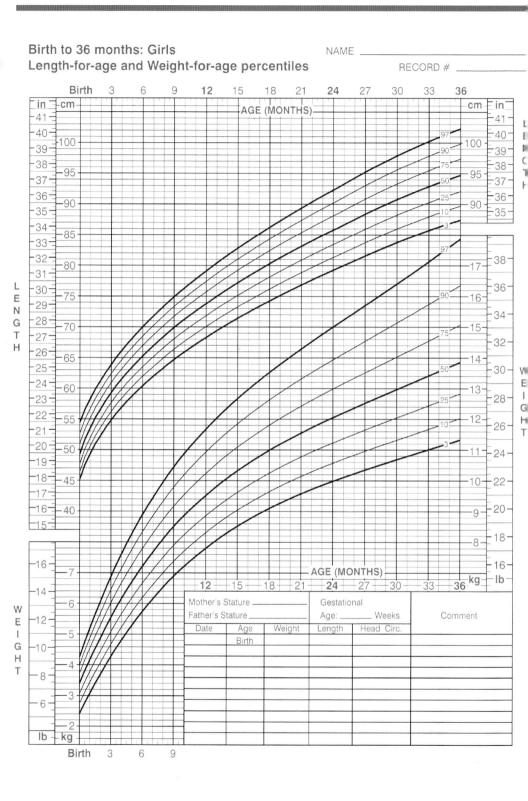

Topics for Mothers of Newborns

TOPICS FOR MOTHERS OF NEWBORNS

37

Bleeding Post-partum

SUMMARY: Some bleeding after birth is normal and to be expected. Generally this is heaviest immediately after the delivery and reduces over time. This normal vaginal discharge after birth is called lochia and is made up of blood cells, uterine lining and bacteria. Due to the significant amount of blood present, it is usually red (lochia rubra). By day 3 or 4, it becomes paler (lochia serosa) and by day 10, it is usually white or yellow-white in colour. Many women also pass small clots of blood during the first few days after delivery. This bleeding may be of greater amounts following a C-section or if the woman experienced vaginal tears or had an episiotomy.

START HERE

- Do you have a fever greater than 38.5°C (101°F) oral / 39°C (102°F) rectal, for at least 24 hours? *or*
- Is bleeding getting heavier (much like a menstrual period)? *or*
- Do you have significant pelvic or abdominal pain? *or*
- Are clots more frequent or getting larger? *or*
- Are you dizzy, light-headed, or feeling faint? *or*
- Did you have low blood (anemia) during pregnancy? *or*
- Does the discharge have a strong foul odour?

YES ▶ **GO TO THE HEALTH CENTRE or HOSPITAL** **H**

NO

See **HOME SUGGESTIONS**

- Is blood loss or discharge improving?

NO ▶ **See Your Doctor**

YES

Continue **HOME SUGGESTIONS**

▶ HOME SUGGESTIONS

1 Get plenty of rest—too much physical activity may cause the bleeding to increase. Normal day-to-day activities are usually well tolerated within 3 or 4 days of delivery, but you should avoid aerobic activity and exercise for 4 to 6 weeks.

2 Take a vitamin supplement with iron.

3 Eat a well-balanced diet, remembering that meat is very high in iron.

4 Drink plenty of fluids: 8 to 10 eight-ounce glasses of water, juice or non-caffeinated soft drinks daily.

5 See the section on **WOUND CARE** (page 42) for other suggestions if you have had a C-Section, vaginal tear or episiotomy.

Mother
Has a Fever after Childbirth

SUMMARY: It is very common for mothers to have a low-grade fever after childbirth: many women will have a temperature of 37.5-38°C transiently over the first 24 hours after delivery which will usually last less than 12 hours. Fevers are especially common if you have had a C-section. High fevers after birth may suggest that a bacterial infection has occurred which will require specific antibiotic therapy. Common sites of infection after delivery include the kidneys, bladder, uterus, fallopian tubes and skin around the vagina. If you had a C-section, episiotomy or tear, the wound may become infected. See the flowchart to help determine if you may have an infection. Several days after delivery some women may develop an infection of the breast called mastitis. As time passes from the time of delivery the less likely an infection will be related to childbirth and more likely that it will represent a common viral infection.

START HERE

BE SURE TO REVIEW THE GENERAL FEVER SECTION PAGE 94

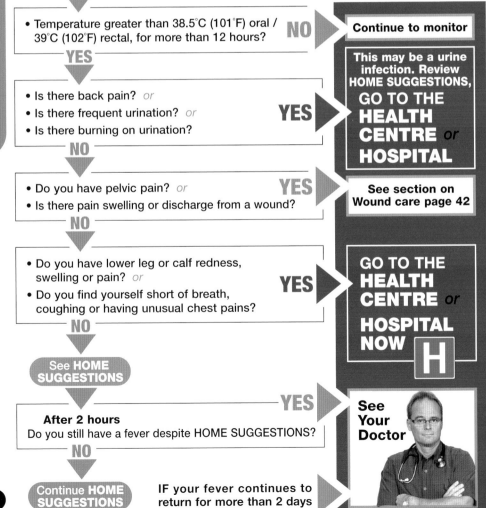

- Temperature greater than 38.5°C (101°F) oral / 39°C (102°F) rectal, for more than 12 hours?

NO → **Continue to monitor**

YES

- Is there back pain? *or*
- Is there frequent urination? *or*
- Is there burning on urination?

YES → **This may be a urine infection. Review HOME SUGGESTIONS, GO TO THE HEALTH CENTRE or HOSPITAL**

NO

- Do you have pelvic pain? *or*
- Is there pain swelling or discharge from a wound?

YES → **See section on Wound care page 42**

NO

- Do you have lower leg or calf redness, swelling or pain? *or*
- Do you find yourself short of breath, coughing or having unusual chest pains?

YES → **GO TO THE HEALTH CENTRE or HOSPITAL NOW** **H**

NO

See **HOME SUGGESTIONS**

After 2 hours
Do you still have a fever despite HOME SUGGESTIONS?

YES → **See Your Doctor**

NO

Continue **HOME SUGGESTIONS**

IF your fever continues to return for more than 2 days

Mother
Has a Fever
after Childbirth

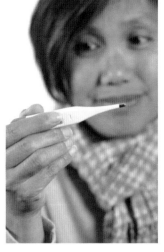

HOME SUGGESTIONS

1 Review the **FEVER** section page 94.
See section on pain medication page 178.

2 Do not overdress. If you feel chills dress warmly but put on dry light clothes when the chills stop.

3 Do not bathe or use cool compresses to bring a temperature down.
This will cause shivering which will actually increase body temperature.

4 Use acetaminophen (**Tylenol** and others) or ibuprofen (**Advil**, **Motrin** and others) for fever and discomfort. See pages 178 for further details.

5 Drink plenty of fluids. You must avoid dehydration. Avoid alcoholic beverages, coffee and regular tea which may make you lose more fluid.

6 Remember fever can be the first sign of a serious illness within days of childbirth. Do not hesitate to consult your doctor. Even if the fever improves with medication, you should see your doctor if you are feeling unwell in other ways.

Care of Your
Episiotomy, Wounds and Vaginal Tears

SUMMARY: During many deliveries there may be tears or an episiotomy, which require repair with stitches to promote healing. Although most experts suggest an episiotomy should be avoided, tears or cuts to the vagina, perineum and vulva are common and must be repaired. Most cesarean sections are now done using the "bikini" cut, which is repaired using stitches or metal clips. Stitches used to repair the birth canal will dissolve and do not need to be removed. The stitches or clips used to close the bikini cut must be removed between 5 and 10 days after delivery. All these wounds generally heal very quickly and completely, though early on they may be quite uncomfortable. The main concerns arise if wounds separate or become infected. If there is no evidence of infection or separation, these wounds can be well managed at home. See the flowchart to assist you in deciding if you need to see your doctor about your wounds.

START HERE

- Do you have a fever greater than 38.5°C (101°F) oral, 39°C (102°F) rectal, for over 24 hours?
    or
- Are the edges of your wound separating?
    or
- Is there bleeding from the wound?
    or
- Is the area around the wound becoming more red or swollen?
    or
- Is there a thick, discoloured discharge from the wound?
    or
- Is there any problem passing urine or stool?

YES ▶ **Take medication for pain or fever (see page 178) and See Your Doctor**

NO ▼

See **HOME SUGGESTIONS**

- Is the wound worse after 8 to 12 hours of treatment?

YES ▶ **See Your Doctor**

NO ▼

Continue **HOME SUGGESTIONS**

and evaluate from the top of this chart every 8 to 12 hours.

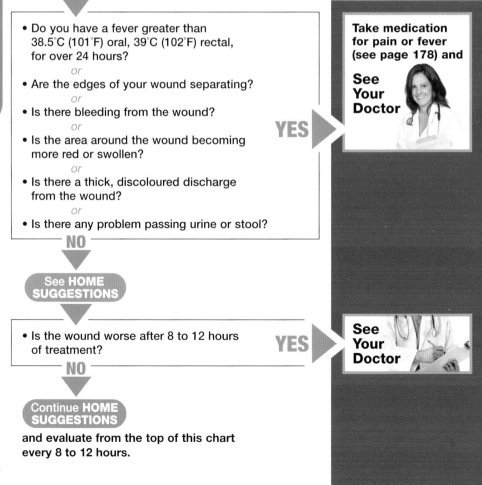

▶HOME SUGGESTIONS

1 Keep the wound clean. It is normal for wounds to have a watery to slightly blood-tinged fluid escaping from the edges as the wound heals. This can be wiped away with warm clean water to avoid a build-up of this material and a crusting over of the wound. Protect the wound from being rubbed against your clothing.

2 Mild swelling can be reduced and controlled with ice—consider laying a bag of frozen peas over your bikini incision. For episiotomy wounds or vaginal tears we suggest you get a gel type freeze pack and place it in a thin cotton cloth or pillow case to apply to the affected area. Apply ice for 10 to 20 minutes as often as every hour or two during the first 24 hours after the repair. Do not apply ice directly to the skin, as it may cause frostbite.

3 After the first couple of days you should switch to the soothing effects of heat to these tender areas. Using a water bottle to spray warm water on the wounds is both soothing and cleansing. Sitz baths in warm water may also be helpful, but should not be taken until 48 hours after delivery.

4 Most wound pain can be treated by using acetaminophen (**Tylenol** and others) or ibuprofen (**Advil**, **Motrin** and others). A combination therapy using acetaminophen with low dose codeine may also helpful. If your pain is more severe you should see your doctor. See page 178 to learn more about pain medication.

5 It is very important to always cleanse the perineum from the front to the back. You must avoid pulling material from the anus over the vaginal area.

6 Some women find that the dry heat provided by a gooseneck lamp aimed at the perineum, but placed no closer than 12 inches, may be soothing.

7 Airing helps. Avoid pads when possible and change them frequently. Do not use tampons until your periods begin again.

After Pains

SUMMARY: Many women will continue to feel pelvic pain that is similar to labour contractions. These cramp-like pains are very common after the second, third and fourth baby. They tend to be stronger and more uncomfortable the more babies a woman has. They are caused by the uterus contracting and are often worse during and after nursing your baby because the same hormone that causes the flow of milk to occur causes these contractions. Most experts believe these pains are "good" as they likely help limit bleeding from the uterus after delivery. No one is going to argue about how they might feel. It is clear that they hurt. Use the flowchart to help decide if you need to see the doctor. Use our **HOME SUGGESTIONS** to reduce your suffering. Fortunately, after pains usually stop by day 3 or 4 after delivery.

START HERE

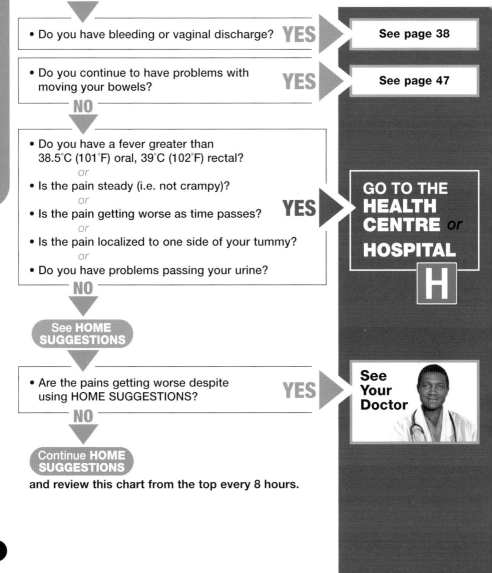

• Do you have bleeding or vaginal discharge? **YES** ▶ **See page 38**

• Do you continue to have problems with moving your bowels? **YES** ▶ **See page 47**

NO

• Do you have a fever greater than 38.5°C (101°F) oral, 39°C (102°F) rectal?
  or
• Is the pain steady (i.e. not crampy)?
  or
• Is the pain getting worse as time passes? **YES** ▶ **GO TO THE HEALTH CENTRE** *or* **HOSPITAL** **H**
  or
• Is the pain localized to one side of your tummy?
  or
• Do you have problems passing your urine?

NO

See **HOME SUGGESTIONS**

• Are the pains getting worse despite using HOME SUGGESTIONS? **YES** ▶ **See Your Doctor**

NO

Continue **HOME SUGGESTIONS**
and review this chart from the top every 8 hours.

▶HOME SUGGESTIONS

1 Most after pains are relieved or at least made more tolerable by using a simple pain medication such as acetaminophen (**Tylenol** and others) or ibuprofen (**Advil**, **Motrin** and others) see page 178. Your doctor may prescribe a combination of acetaminophen and codeine if the acetaminophen is not adequate by itself. Watch out for constipation if you take codeine. See page 47 to help manage constipation.

2 Too much activity can worsen crampy after pains. Normal activity is usually possible by day 3 to 4 after a vaginal delivery and by day 7 after a C-section or vaginal delivery with significant tears or an episiotomy.

3 Avoiding problems with passing your urine or stool will lessen pelvic or abdominal discomfort (see **MOTHER IS CONSTIPATED** page 47). A regular diet which is high in fibre and 8 to 10 glasses of water per day should help.

4 A hot water bottle or warm bath will often help ease cramps.

5 It is very common to feel an increase in pain when nursing so you should take some pain medication 20 to 30 minutes prior to breast-feeding.

6 During the first few days after delivery we suggest that you try to take your pain medication on a regular schedule to reduce after pains. If you wait until the pain gets really bad then the medication will not help as much. You should take acetaminophen every 4 to 6 hours or ibuprofen every 6 to 8 hours.

AFTER PAINS

Breast Pain

SUMMARY: The most common cause of breast pain or tenderness after delivery is engorgement because the breasts are full of milk. Feeding or expressing milk may relieve this breast fullness. There are other causes of breast pain which are more serious. Breasts that are red, locally tender to the touch or if you have fever in association with sore, tender red breasts may suggest infection. Use the flowchart to help decide if you should see your doctor.

START HERE

BREAST PAIN

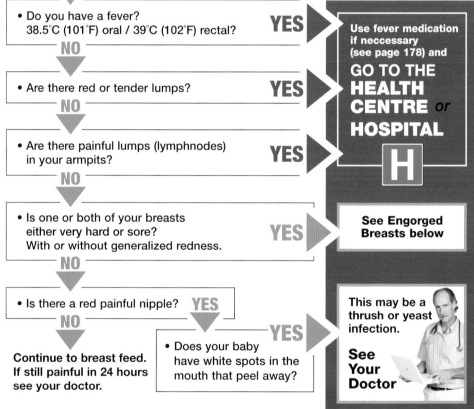

- Do you have a fever?
  38.5°C (101°F) oral / 39°C (102°F) rectal? **YES**

  NO

- Are there red or tender lumps? **YES**

  NO

- Are there painful lumps (lymphnodes) in your armpits? **YES**

  NO

Use fever medication if neccessary (see page 178) and

GO TO THE HEALTH CENTRE or **HOSPITAL**

H

- Is one or both of your breasts either very hard or sore? With or without generalized redness. **YES**

  NO

See Engorged Breasts below

- Is there a red painful nipple? **YES**

  NO

Continue to breast feed. If still painful in 24 hours see your doctor.

- Does your baby have white spots in the mouth that peel away? **YES**

This may be a thrush or yeast infection.

See Your Doctor

ENGORGED BREASTS

Engorgement or a breast full of milk that cannot drain is usually due to a blocked milk duct not infection. The breast is usually very firm to feel and may be generally red all over. To treat this condition, soak in a warm tub with the breasts submerged. Continue to breast-feed from the painful breast, starting from the worst breast first. Take acetaminophen (**Tylenol** or others) for the pain (see pain medication page 178). Try to express milk manually or with an electric breast pump after feeding. If baby cannot latch because of the firmness of the breasts, express some milk before feeding.

If this advice does not improve your situation within 24 hours or if the breasts are becoming more red or swollen, please see your doctor.

If you decide to bottle-feed your baby with formula, some degree of breast engorgement is likely. You can minimize this by trying to limit stimulation or movement of your breasts using a snug-fitting bra. Following our suggestions above for minor engorgement is useful. In the past, doctors prescribed drugs to prevent milk production but these prescription drugs are no longer considered safe.

Mother is Constipated

SUMMARY: Constipation (difficulty in passing stools) is not a common problem after delivery unless it was also a problem before pregnancy. Many women do experience some difficulty with bowel activity late in pregnancy which may be due to a lack of space in the pelvis as the baby "drops" into position. New mothers may not move their bowel for 2 to 3 days after delivery which is normal though it may be interpreted as constipation. There are several reasons for the reduction in bowel activity: first, the lower bowel usually empties during labour and delivery; secondly, most women do not eat much during labour and delivery; thirdly, normal eating does not resume for 2 to 4 hours after delivery and may be delayed further if anaesthesia was used. This delay in bowel activity may be compounded by a tendency for some women to hold back from moving their bowels due to the fear of pain associated with the swelling of the perineum. Using a high insoluble fibre diet with plenty of liquids can help maintain normal bowel activity. Follow the flowchart to determine if you should be seeing your doctor about constipation.

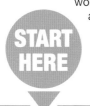

START HERE

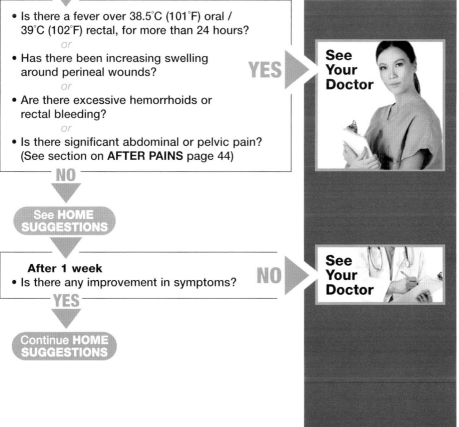

- Is there a fever over 38.5°C (101°F) oral / 39°C (102°F) rectal, for more than 24 hours?
  or
- Has there been increasing swelling around perineal wounds?
  or
- Are there excessive hemorrhoids or rectal bleeding?
  or
- Is there significant abdominal or pelvic pain? (See section on **AFTER PAINS** page 44)

YES → **See Your Doctor**

NO

See **HOME SUGGESTIONS**

After 1 week
- Is there any improvement in symptoms?

NO → **See Your Doctor**

YES

Continue **HOME SUGGESTIONS**

▶ HOME SUGGESTIONS

1   It is normal to miss bowel movements for one or two days after delivery.
A return to your normal diet will often bring a return to the previous bowel habits.
Often new mothers "forget" to eat due to fatigue and being busy looking after a
new baby. Don't forget to look after yourself too!

2   Keeping stools soft will make that first bowel movement easier to pass.
Most new mothers are pleasantly surprised that the first bowel movement is
not as uncomfortable as anticipated when the stools are soft. As good way
to ensure soft stools is to have 1 to 2 tablespoons of a psyllium product
(**Metamucil**, **Prodiem** and others) daily starting the day after delivery.
Be sure to take these fibre supplements with at least 8 to 10 oz of fluid
with each dose.

3   Sometimes excessive swelling due to hemorrhoids or wound healing
(see section on **CARE OF WOUNDS** page 42) may make bowel movements
more difficult. If stools are soft this is not so much of a problem. If pain or
swelling continues to be a problem, then you should see your doctor.

4   Using an over-the-counter laxative on a regular basis is generally not a
good idea. However, if getting a bowel movement started seems to be the
problem then we would recommend a glycerin suppository. Enemas should be
avoided until wounds are healed. **Milk of Magnesia** (30cc or 2 tablespoons)
may also be helpful and can be taken once or twice daily as it is less harsh
than laxatives containing senna.

Leg Pains and Cramps

SUMMARY: Throughout the latter part of pregnancy, during labour and after delivery, leg cramps or pain are common, usually in the lower leg. Sometimes this discomfort is due to varicose veins which, although a nuisance, are not usually serious. Occasionally, however, leg cramps or pains can be a sign of a more serious problem such as blood clots or thrombophlebitis. This more serious condition needs to be assessed by a physician. Use the flowchart to help you decide if you should see the doctor.

START HERE

In addition to leg pain or cramps do you have:
• The discomfort in only one leg?
  or
• Swelling of one calf or ankle in comparison to the other?
  or
• Redness and warmth to touch the calf?
  or
• Tenderness of the calf even when there is no cramping?

YES → See Your Doctor

NO

See **HOME SUGGESTIONS**

Review your leg symptoms and review this chart 2 or 3 times daily

• Are your symptoms getting worse? **YES** → See Your Doctor

NO

Continue **HOME SUGGESTIONS**

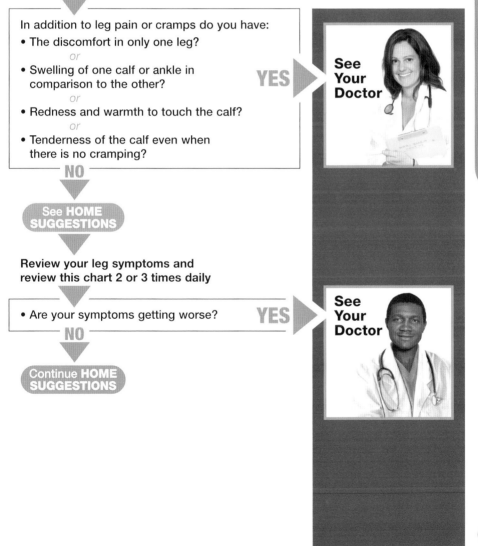

▶ HOME SUGGESTIONS

1 What causes leg cramping is poorly understood. It may be that during delivery the muscles are either used more or in an unusual way and this physical exercise has caused the muscle to be sore simply due to unusual exertion. Rest, gentle massage, local heat and some pain medication may relieve this pain. See page 178 about the use of pain medication.

2 A well-balanced diet providing adequate amounts of potassium and calcium is important for normal muscle function.

3 Passive stretching of the calves (gently pulling your toes towards your face from the ankle) will provide relief from cramps. Regular stretching may prevent cramps from starting.

4 Simple analgesics such acetaminophen (**Tylenol** and others) or ibuprofen (**Advil**, **Motrin** and others) often control persistent pain due to cramping.

5 Non-prescription muscle relaxants are usually not very effective in relieving cramps and are not recommended when breast-feeding.

Birth Control and Sexual Health

SUMMARY: There are no hard and fast rules about when couples should start to have sexual intercourse again after childbirth: only about one-third of women have intercourse during the first 6 weeks after delivery and about 40% of women who engage in sexual activity before 12 weeks will have some pain or discomfort. Minor vaginal tears and lacerations will heal 2 or 3 weeks after delivery. Because there is some risk of infection if sexual relations begin before 3 weeks, we recommend that you not consider sexual intercourse until after 2 or 3 weeks. Breast-feeding may cause some vaginal dryness due to the low estrogen levels that occur during breast-feeding. Many couples are too tired to have sex due to the demands of the new baby and as a result of the ever-changing schedule that the baby brings, but the most important consideration is the woman's comfort and desire.

Periods often return within 6 to 8 weeks after breast-feeding stops but can occur as early as 4 weeks after delivery even if you are nursing. Breast-feeding is not an adequate form of birth control. Ovulation and hence the ability to become pregnant again is just as variable. As a result couples will have to practice birth control if an early pregnancy is not desired.

Women who are breast-feeding should not take the birth control pill until breast-feeding is well established.

See the flowchart to help decide the kind of birth control which is right for you.

IF YOUR FAMILY IS COMPLETE

• Do you wish permanent sterilization? **YES**

NO

> **Consider tubal ligation for women** or **Consider a vasectomy for men. Please discuss with your doctor**

TEMPORARY CONTRACEPTION

If you are not sure your family is complete you should consider temporary contraception

• Are you breast-feeding? **NO**

YES

> **Use barrier method - condom, diaphragm** (only after 6 weeks) or **Hormonal - oral birth control pill, progestin injections or implant**

• Is breast-feeding well established? **NO**

YES

> **Use barrier method - condom, diaphragm** (only after 6 weeks)

Consider using barrier method - condom, diaphragm (only after 6 weeks) or **Consider using an IUD** (intrauterine device) or **Hormonal - oral birth control pill, progestin injections or implant**

See **HOME SUGGESTIONS**

▶ HOME SUGGESTIONS

1 The birth control pill is usually safe for nursing mothers who are otherwise able to take hormonal contraception once breast-feeding is established. It may, however, decrease milk production and if this is significant, the pill should be stopped and another form of birth control should be used. The "progestin" only methods (injection and implants) may have less effect on milk production. Discuss these issues with you doctor at a routine visit.

2 Using a diaphragm after childbirth may be a problem because the diaphragm that you used before becoming pregnant may no longer fit. The fit should be checked by your doctor before you depend on this method of birth control. As time passes, the diaphragm will likely fit better. Usually after 6 weeks healing is complete.

3 The rhythm method is not a reliable form of birth control after childbirth as the return of ovulation is variable and unpredictable.

4 Spermicidal agents should be used with condoms. This will prevent unwanted pregnancy if the condom leaks or breaks.

5 The decision to undergo a procedure like tubal ligation or vasectomy should be considered permanent and irreversible.

The Post-partum Blues or Depression

SUMMARY: It is very common for new mothers to experience a low mood or mild depression after childbirth. This is usually a temporary problem but can become a serious medical condition requiring treatment if it lasts. There are many reasons for this change in mood which include: fatigue from loss of sleep; the uncertainty related to caring for a new baby; the discomfort after delivery; and the emotional letdown after anticipation and fear of labour and delivery. Most mothers experience all of these feelings to some degree. The mood changes may develop as early as 2 to 4 days after delivery and in some women, may persist for up to 2 weeks. You should not be alarmed if your depressed mood seems to be lasting much longer. Studies have shown that this depression may last as long as 18 months.

It is natural to feel guilty about these feelings of depression when everyone else seems so happy about the new baby. Unfortunately this guilt tends to make the depression worse. It may be helpful to share your feelings with others. Sometimes medication can help. Depression is now recognized as a chemical imbalance and can be corrected. Don't be afraid to tell your doctor about how you are feeling. Often doctors forget to ask about depression in women after delivery.

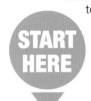

START HERE

• Have you fears of harming yourself, your child or another person?

YES ▶

NO ▼

• Do you experience periods of feeling "blue" / low mood?
  or
• Are you crying spontaneously for no reason?
  or
• Do you lack interest or have trouble "getting going"?
  or
• Is your fatigue excessive?
  or
• Is your appetite up or down in comparison to normal?
  or
• Is your sleep disturbed or not refreshing?

YES ▶

After 7 to 10 days
• Are you still feeling the same "blue" symptoms?

YES ▶

NO ▼

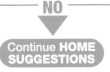
Continue **HOME SUGGESTIONS**

GO TO THE HEALTH CENTRE or HOSPITAL

H

See next page
▶ HOME SUGGESTIONS

and discuss these feelings with your doctor on the next visit.

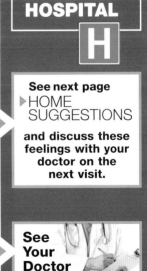
See Your Doctor

POST-PARTUM BLUES

53

The Post-partum
Blues or Depression

▶ HOME SUGGESTIONS

1 A change in mood after the delivery of your child is normal. You do not have to feel guilty if you are feeling the blues. You should try to discuss your feelings with your partner, family, close friends and your doctor. Be assured that these feelings usually resolve themselves, but even if they don't there is treatment available. You should discuss this with your doctor.

2 Get your rest. Although this may sound crazy with all the demands of a new baby it is possible and often means letting other things go for a short time. Try to rest whenever the baby is sleeping. Don't hesitate to ask for or accept help from others.

3 Eat properly. Often with all the care the new baby takes, new mothers don't make time to look after their own nutritional needs.

4 Do some light to moderate exercise. A brisk short walk takes only a short time but is worth it. This exercise time is a bit of time for yourself. It burns excess adrenaline and allows dad to have some time alone with the new baby!

5 Use pain medication (see page 178) to treat the discomforts that occur after delivery. These medications are safe even if you are breast-feeding. You'll feel better about yourself if you are more comfortable.

6 Try to relax and not be concerned that everything must be perfect. There is no "right way" to do things with your baby. Experimentation and time will sort out most things so that you can enjoy these early weeks and months.

7 Avoid non-prescription treatments for depression. If your mood does not improve or you feel worse be sure to talk to your doctor. Sometimes a prescription medication may be necessary and is safe even if you are breast-feeding.

Topics for Children

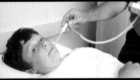
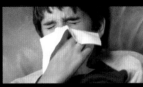
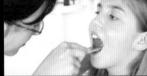
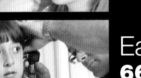
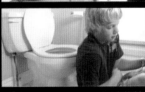
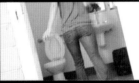
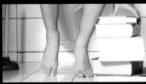
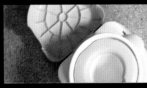
TOPICS FOR CHILDREN

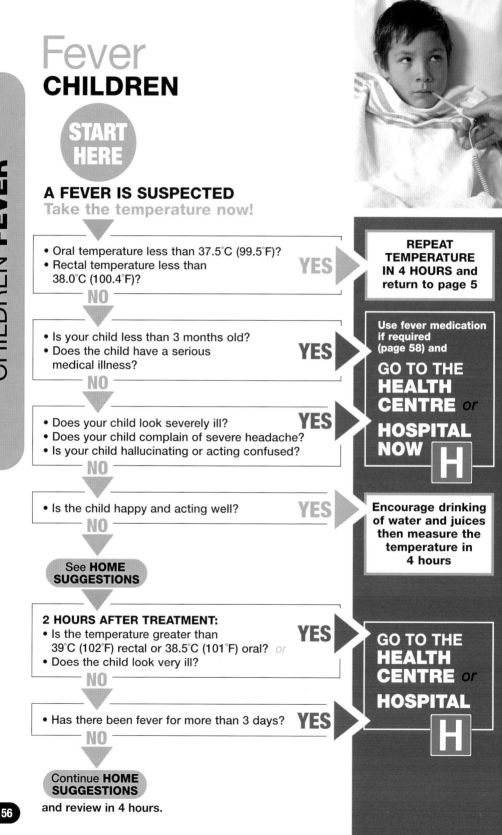

Fever
CHILDREN

START HERE

A FEVER IS SUSPECTED
Take the temperature now!

- Oral temperature less than 37.5°C (99.5°F)?
- Rectal temperature less than 38.0°C (100.4°F)?

YES → **REPEAT TEMPERATURE IN 4 HOURS and return to page 5**

NO

- Is your child less than 3 months old?
- Does the child have a serious medical illness?

YES → Use fever medication if required (page 58) and **GO TO THE HEALTH CENTRE** *or* **HOSPITAL NOW** **H**

NO

- Does your child look severely ill?
- Does your child complain of severe headache?
- Is your child hallucinating or acting confused?

YES →

NO

- Is the child happy and acting well?

YES → Encourage drinking of water and juices then measure the temperature in 4 hours

NO

See **HOME SUGGESTIONS**

2 HOURS AFTER TREATMENT:
- Is the temperature greater than 39°C (102°F) rectal or 38.5°C (101°F) oral? *or*
- Does the child look very ill?

YES → **GO TO THE HEALTH CENTRE** *or* **HOSPITAL** **H**

NO

- Has there been fever for more than 3 days? **YES**

NO

Continue **HOME SUGGESTIONS**
and review in 4 hours.

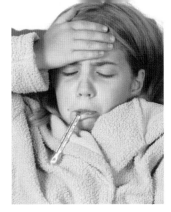

▶HOME
SUGGESTIONS

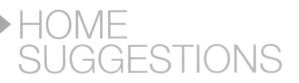

1   When your child has a fever, dress the child lightly and don't cover with blankets.

2   If the child starts to shiver, dress them warmly until it stops, then dress lightly again.

3   Give acetaminophen (**Tylenol** and others) every 4 hours if the child is uncomfortable or if the child's temperature is high (see chart on page 58 for proper dose). Ibuprofen (**Advil**, **Motrin** and others) may be used instead of acetaminophen. Ibuprofen is taken every 6 to 8 hours. Do not use ASA (**Aspirin** and others) in anyone under 20 years of age (see page 178).

4   If the child vomits the medication given for pain or fever, you can use acetaminophen suppositories (medication given rectally) instead. Ask your pharmacist for help.

5   We suggest that you do not sponge bath your feverish child. Sponge baths tend to reduce the temperature for only a short time and make many children unhappy and uncomfortable. Bathing may also cause shivering which will raise the temperature again.

6   Encourage the child to drink plenty of liquids. Fluid losses are increased with fever.

7   Take the temperature every 4 hours and certainly if you feel the fever is worse.

8   If the child complains of a sore throat, cough, earache or other problems, please review these topics as well.

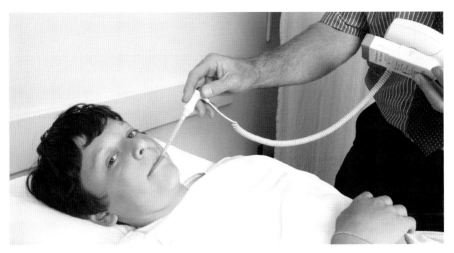

Medication information

Acetaminophen dosing chart

Using an age chart to decide upon dosage will always underdose heavier children in the age group. If you are comfortable with doing some basic math you can figure out a precise dose for your child if you know their weight. Physicians decide whether or not a proper dose has been given by multiplying the child's weight in kilograms by 15, or the weight in pounds by 6.5. This gives the total milligrams of acetaminophen that is needed per dose. You then can choose the dose of liquid or number of tablets needed from the chart below.

For example: A child weighs 20 lbs X 6.5 mg/lb = 130 mg.
This may be rounded down to 120 mg for a convenient dose.
You should check the dosage calculated before giving this to your child.

WEIGHT		DOSE	80 mg/1 ml 5 ml=1 tsp	160 mg/5 ml	80 mg tabs	160 mg tabs Junior	325 mg tabs Regular	500 mg tabs X-strength
Pounds	Kilograms							
7-10 lbs	<5 kg	40 mg	.5 ml	1.25 ml	1/2 tab			
10-18 lbs	5-8 kg	80 mg	1.0 ml	2.5 ml	1 tab	1/2 tab		
18-26 lbs	8-12 kg	120 mg	1.5 ml		1 1/2 tabs			
26-35 lbs	12-16 kg	160 mg	2.0 ml	5.0 ml	2 tabs	1 tab	1/2 tab	
35-45 lbs	16-20 kg	240 mg	3.0 ml	7.5 ml	3 tabs	1 1/2 tabs		
45-55 lbs	20-25 kg	320 mg	4.0 ml	10.0 ml	4 tabs	2 tabs	1 tab	
55-65 lbs	25-30 kg	400 mg	5.0 ml	12.5 ml	5 tabs	2 1/2 tabs		
65-80 lbs	30-36 kg	480 mg		15.0 ml	6 tabs	3 tabs	1 1/2 tabs	1 tab
80-95 lbs	36-44 kg	560 mg		17.5 ml	7 tabs	3 1/2 tabs	1 3/4 tabs	1 tab
95-145 lbs	44-65 kg	650 mg				4 tabs	2 tabs	1 1/2 tabs
145 lbs +	65 kg +	650-1000 mg					2-3 tabs	2 tabs

Use the weight chart and go across to find the most convenient form of acetaminophen. This will help you choose which type to purchase.

Ibuprofen dosing chart

As outlined in the acetaminophen chart instructions, the dose of ibuprofen should depend on the individual's weight. If you use age as the determinant of dose, you will underdose all the larger children in that age group. The dose of ibuprofen is 10 mg per kilogram (2 lbs) of body weight and can be given every 6 to 8 hours.

WEIGHT		DOSE	80 mg/1 ml 5 ml=1 tsp	200 mg tabs
Pounds	Kilograms			
7-10 lbs	<5 kg	40 mg	2 ml or 1/2 tsp	
10-18 lbs	5-8 kg	60 mg	3 ml or 1/2 tsp	
18-25 lbs	8-12 kg	100 mg	5 ml or 1 tsp	1/2 tab
26-30 lbs	12-14 kg	140 mg	7 ml or 1 1/2 tsp	3/4 tab
30-35 lbs	14-16 kg	150 mg	8 ml or 1 1/2 tsp	3/4 tab
35-45 lbs	16-20 kg	170 mg	9 ml or 1 3/4 tsp	3/4 tab
45-55 lbs	20-25 kg	200 mg	10 ml or 2 tsp	1 tab
55-75 lbs	25-35 kg	300 mg	15 ml or 3 tsp	1 1/2 tab
75-125 lbs	35-60 kg	400 mg	20 ml or 4 tsp	2 tabs
125-150 lbs	60-70 kg	up to 600 mg		up to 3 tabs
150-200 lbs	70-90 kg	up to 800 mg		up to 4 tabs
200 lbs +	90 kg +	up to 800 mg		4 tabs

Cough & Cold
and "the Flu"

SUMMARY: First of all, it is important to understand that the average child gets 6 to 10 colds per year. Many of these colds may be mild and go unnoticed by parents. Colds are caused by viruses. **Antibiotics will have no effect on the viruses that cause colds.** The symptoms of a cold can be treated very successfully at home. While having a sick child at home can be distressing, most children with colds do not need to see a physician.

Occasional vomiting, or throwing up, after a coughing spell is common and is not a serious symptom. A cold may cause a dry cough which can last up to 2 or 3 weeks after other symptoms have passed. Sore throats and earaches are also commonly associated with colds (see pages 63 and 66).

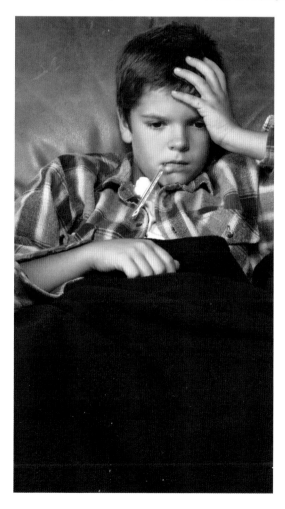

CHILDREN
Possible Symptoms:

- ▸ runny nose
- ▸ congested nose
- ▸ cough
- ▸ swollen glands
- ▸ sore throat
- ▸ sore ears
- ▸ watery eyes
- ▸ cough
- ▸ fever
- ▸ irritability
- ▸ reduced appetite
- ▸ interrupted sleep

Cough & Cold and "the Flu"

CHILDREN

START HERE

COMMON COLD SYMPTOMS

- Is your child less than 3 months old?
  or
- Does your child have a fever above 38.5°C (101°F) oral / 39°C (102°F) rectal?
  or
- Does the child look severely ill?
  or
- Does your child have difficulty breathing?
  or
- Does your child have severe difficulty swallowing?

NO

YES ▶ Use fever medication if required (page 58) and **GO TO THE HEALTH CENTRE** *or* **HOSPITAL NOW** Ⓗ

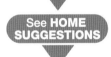
See **HOME SUGGESTIONS**

- Has there been a fever greater than 37.5°C (99.5°F) oral / 38°C (100.4°F) rectal for more than 3 days?
  or
- Is there poor intake of fluids?
  or
- Is the nose discharge consistently green?
  or
- Is the child coughing up green coloured sputum?

NO

YES ▶ **GO TO THE HEALTH CENTRE** *or* **HOSPITAL** Ⓗ

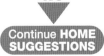
Continue **HOME SUGGESTIONS**

Reassess your child from the top of this chart every 4 hours.

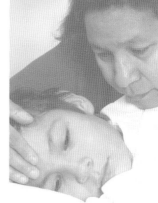

Cough & Cold
and "the Flu"
CHILDREN

► HOME SUGGESTIONS

Remember, there is no cure for the common cold.
Antibiotics will not shorten the cold or cure it.

You can, however, help your child to feel better by following these suggestions:

1   If your child has a fever see the **FEVER** section on pages 56-57.

2   Use acetaminophen (**Tylenol** and others) or ibuprofen (**Advil**, **Motrin** and others) to control fever and relieve discomfort. See page 58 for acetaminophen dosage. ASA (**Aspirin** and others) should not be given to anyone under 20 years of age with a viral illness. See page 178 for an explanation.

3   For a runny nose: If your child is able, encourage them to blow their nose. Don't discourage sniffing. It's actually a good way to clear the nose and does not push infection into the ears or sinuses.
For very young children who cannot blow and clear their nose themselves, use a rubber bulb to gently suction out mucus.
A saline nasal spray, purchased from your pharmacy, can help dry the nose. Do not use decongestant nasal sprays for children.

4   For a plugged nose: While your child is lying on their back, drip 3 drops of warm tap water in each nostril. After 1 minute, have the child blow their nose or use the bulb suction as described above. Repeat as often as necessary.

5   Oral decongestant medication or combination medications, like **Dimetapp**, can help dry up a runny nose and improve sleep (see page 176). However, do not use decongestant medications where there is severe heart disease, poorly controlled high blood pressure or severe asthma. Antihistamines are not recommended for children under 2 years.

6   Cough syrups with "DM" (dextromethorphan) may be helpful for a dry cough if getting to sleep or concentrating at school is a problem. You don't want to suppress a wet or loose cough because this type of cough is clearing the mucus from the chest. "DM" should not be given to a child if they are having breathing problems (e.g. asthma or croup). Do not give "DM" to children under 1 year.

7   Sipping warm drinks can help loosen a cough. Warm water with sugar or warm juice such as lemonade, or chicken soup are good examples.

continued next page...

Cough & Cold and "the Flu"
CHILDREN

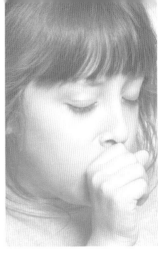

▶ # HOME SUGGESTIONS

8 A lozenge may help a sore and dry throat if the child is old enough to have a hard candy. Choose a flavour that your child likes. Expensive lozenges are not necessary as hard candies of any kind work well.

9 Do not expose your child to cigarette smoke.

10 Your child should not exercise or play hard, and should get plenty of rest. Make sure they drink extra fluids. Use a cool mist humidifier in your home if you have one.

11 **Do not stop breast-feeding.** Feed your child smaller portions more often if necessary.

12 Frequent handwashing can decrease the spread of infection.

Sore Throat

SUMMARY: Keep in mind that sore throats are a common childhood problem. Viral infections (the common cold) are often the cause of the sore throat. Most sore throats **DO NOT RESPOND TO ANTIBIOTICS**. The pain and discomfort will usually ease within 48 hours and many sore throats will feel better after some simple therapy at home. Follow the flowchart to help you decide if you should take your child to the doctor.

CHILDREN
Possible Symptoms:

▶ pain in the throat
▶ difficulty swallowing
▶ refusal to eat and drink
▶ fever
▶ red throat or pus on the tonsils
▶ swollen glands in the neck
▶ other cold symptoms

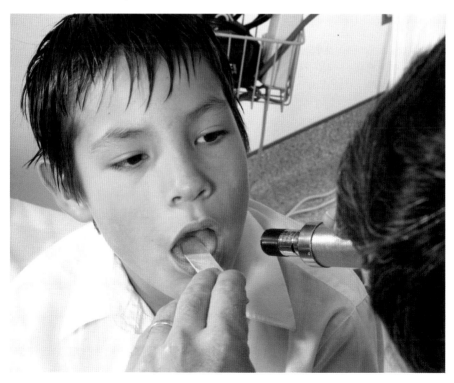

Sore Throat
CHILDREN

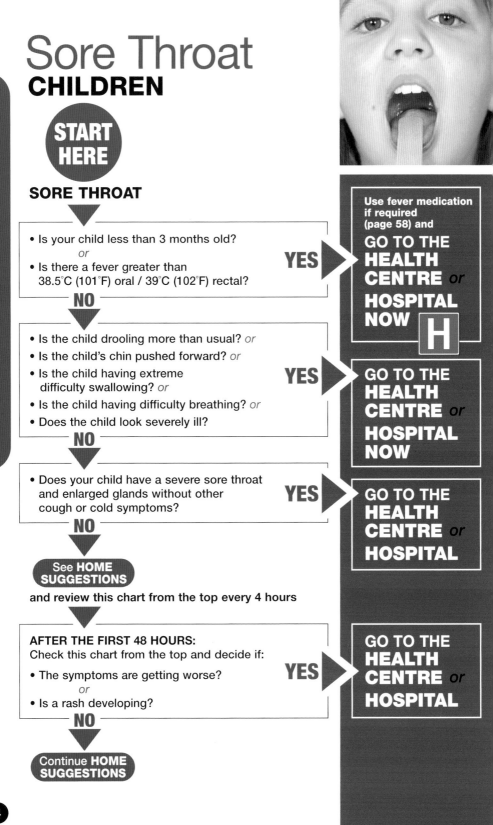

START HERE

SORE THROAT

- Is your child less than 3 months old? *or*
- Is there a fever greater than 38.5°C (101°F) oral / 39°C (102°F) rectal?

YES ➤ Use fever medication if required (page 58) and **GO TO THE HEALTH CENTRE** or **HOSPITAL NOW** **H**

NO

- Is the child drooling more than usual? *or*
- Is the child's chin pushed forward? *or*
- Is the child having extreme difficulty swallowing? *or*
- Is the child having difficulty breathing? *or*
- Does the child look severely ill?

YES ➤ **GO TO THE HEALTH CENTRE** or **HOSPITAL NOW**

NO

- Does your child have a severe sore throat and enlarged glands without other cough or cold symptoms?

YES ➤ **GO TO THE HEALTH CENTRE** or **HOSPITAL**

NO

See HOME SUGGESTIONS

and review this chart from the top every 4 hours

AFTER THE FIRST 48 HOURS:
Check this chart from the top and decide if:

- The symptoms are getting worse? *or*
- Is a rash developing?

YES ➤ **GO TO THE HEALTH CENTRE** or **HOSPITAL**

NO

Continue HOME SUGGESTIONS

Sore Throat
CHILDREN

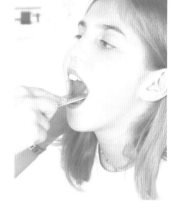

▶ HOME SUGGESTIONS

1 If your child has a fever with a sore throat please see the **FEVER** section on page 56.

2 You may give your child acetaminophen (**Tylenol** and others) or ibuprofen (**Advil**, **Motrin** and others) for pain. See page 58 for acetaminophen dosage. See page 178 for further information and advice about pain medication. ASA (**Aspirin** and others) should not be given to anyone 20 years and younger.

3 Make sure your child has plenty of cool drinks which will help soothe the throat.

4 Gargles or anesthetic preparations can help reduce the pain of a sore throat and make eating less troublesome. A salt water gargle (1/2 to 1 teaspoon of salt in 8 oz of warm water) may give some relief and can be used several times daily. Younger children may have trouble gargling and if they tend to swallow the mixture, reduce the salt content to 1/4 to 1/2 teaspoon. Avoid gargling at all if it is too painful, or if the child cannot gargle without choking.
You can buy local anesthetic ("freezing" or "numbing") sprays (**Chloraseptic**) and gargles at your pharmacy. These medicines usually contain 0.5% phenol and a flavouring. We have found that children may eat more comfortably if these sprays are used before meals. Swallowing one or two tablespoons of corn syrup may also soothe a sore throat.

5 For children over age 1 year, give a teaspoon of honey 3 times daily. **DO NOT GIVE HONEY TO CHILDREN UNDER 1 YEAR OF AGE.**

6 If your child is old enough to have a hard candy, allow them to suck on a lozenge. One does not have to buy expensive lozenges. Hard candies of almost any kind will work well.

7 Give your child plenty to drink. Children may find it more comfortable to swallow soft foods and soups for the first few days.

8 Frequent handwashing can decrease the spread of infection.

Earache

SUMMARY: You can have an ear infection which occurs outside the ear drum in the ear canal or behind the ear drum. Ear canal infections may develop after a day of swimming or water play ("swimmer's ear"). Similarly, the ear canal is more likely to become infected if it has been irritated by using cotton swabs.

Infections behind the ear drum, called middle ear infections, can result from congestion during a cold or flu when the Eustachian tube plugs and the normal drainage to the throat is blocked. Middle ear infections are uncommon in children under 6 months of age. Breast-fed babies seem to have fewer ear infections.

CHILDREN
Possible Symptoms:

▸ earache
▸ poor hearing
▸ drainage from the ear
▸ fever
▸ sore glands around the ear or in the neck
▸ pain when the ear is tugged
▸ itchy ears
▸ infants may pull on their ear

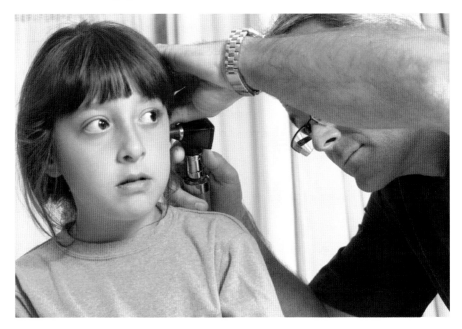

Earache
CHILDREN

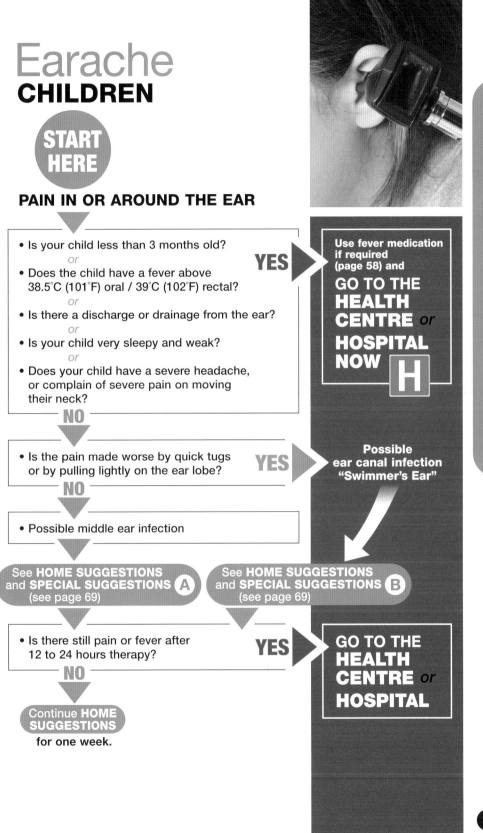

START HERE

PAIN IN OR AROUND THE EAR

▼

- Is your child less than 3 months old?
  or
- Does the child have a fever above 38.5°C (101°F) oral / 39°C (102°F) rectal?
  or
- Is there a discharge or drainage from the ear?
  or
- Is your child very sleepy and weak?
  or
- Does your child have a severe headache, or complain of severe pain on moving their neck?

YES ▶ Use fever medication if required (page 58) and **GO TO THE HEALTH CENTRE or HOSPITAL NOW** **H**

NO ▼

- Is the pain made worse by quick tugs or by pulling lightly on the ear lobe?

YES ▶ Possible ear canal infection "Swimmer's Ear"

NO ▼

- Possible middle ear infection

See **HOME SUGGESTIONS** and **SPECIAL SUGGESTIONS** **A** (see page 69)

See **HOME SUGGESTIONS** and **SPECIAL SUGGESTIONS** **B** (see page 69)

- Is there still pain or fever after 12 to 24 hours therapy?

YES ▶ **GO TO THE HEALTH CENTRE or HOSPITAL**

NO ▼

Continue **HOME SUGGESTIONS** for one week.

CHILDREN **EARACHE**

67

Earache
CHILDREN

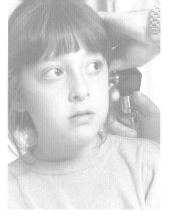

▶ HOME
SUGGESTIONS

1 If your child has a fever, please see the **FEVER** section on page 56.

2 Give your child acetaminophen (**Tylenol** and others) or Ibuprofen (**Advil**, **Motrin** and others) for pain. See page 178 for more details about pain medication. See page 58 for acetaminophen dosage. Do not use ASA (**Aspirin** and others) in anyone under 20 years of age (see page 178 for an explanation).

3 Your child can be made more comfortable by putting a warm cloth on the ear for 20 minutes several times daily.

4 Sometimes putting warm oil drops in the ear canal may give some relief. You can buy **Auralgan** drops or simply use mineral oil, cooking oil or olive oil. Heat the oil in warm water. Do not boil the water. Make sure you test the temperature of the oil drops on your skin before placing it in your child's ear.

5 If you are breast-feeding, do not stop, but try to nurse so the child is in an upright position. If necessary feed smaller amounts more often.

6 Do not expose your child to cigarette smoke.

7 Read about **FEVER**, **COUGH AND COLD**, and **SORE THROAT** if necessary.

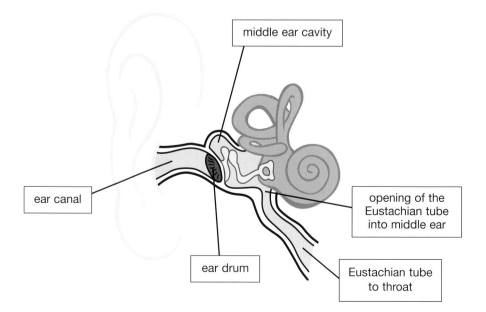

middle ear cavity

ear canal

opening of the Eustachian tube into middle ear

ear drum

Eustachian tube to throat

Earache
CHILDREN

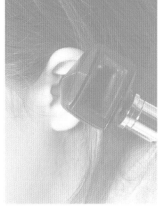

▶ HOME SUGGESTIONS

SPECIAL SUGGESTIONS (A)
When your child has middle ear pain:

1. Encourage your child to "pop" their ears by blowing against a pinched nose. Have them do this several times daily.

2. Doctors now know that most middle ear infections do not need to be treated with antibiotics. Use pain medication early. Night-time visits to the emergency department are usually unnecessary.

3. Repeated ear infections may be prevented. Ask your family doctor.

SPECIAL SUGGESTIONS (B)
When your child has an ear canal infection or "Swimmer's Ear":

1. Keep the child's ear dry for at least 7 days. Avoid swimming or water play that involves getting water in the ears. A few drops of a drying agent will help the ear dry faster. **Buro-sol** or a mixture of 1 tablespoon of vinegar in 1 tablespoon of warm water makes a good drying agent.

2. This is an infection which may improve with the non-prescription antibiotic drop (**Polysporin**). Use 2 drops 4 times daily.

3. **DO NOT TRY TO CLEAN THE EAR OUT OR PUT OBJECTS, SUCH AS COTTON SWABS, INTO THE EAR.**

4. If your child gets infections of the ear canal repeatedly you may want to try and prevent these before symptoms appear. Placing a couple of drops of cooking, olive or mineral oil in the canal before swimming or placing a couple of drops of antibiotic solution (**Polysporin**) in the canal after a day of swimming may help to prevent repeat infections.

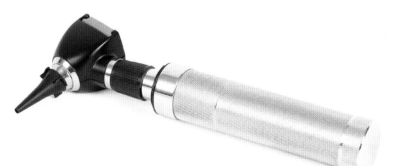

Vomiting or "the Stomach Flu"

SUMMARY: Vomiting, or "throwing up", is the forceful exit of your stomach contents by way of the mouth. Infants often spit up, but in a gentle way; this is different from vomiting. The most common cause of vomiting is the "stomach flu", a viral illness. You can usually care for your child by changing their diet and letting the symptoms run their course. Your child will not usually require medication to treat the "stomach flu". If you can keep your child drinking small amounts frequently, you should not need to see your doctor. This is especially true if the child looks well between episodes of vomiting.

CHILDREN

Possible Symptoms:

▸ vomiting ("throwing up")

And some or all of the following:

▸ abdominal pain   ▸ fever

▸ cramps   ▸ diarrhea

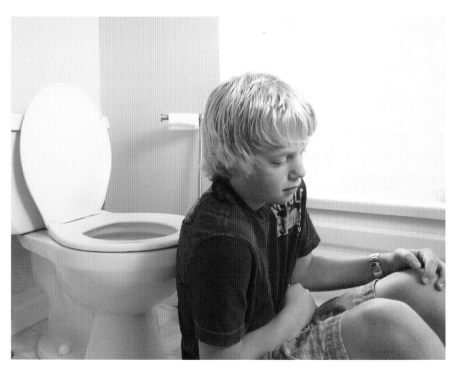

Vomiting or "the Stomach Flu"
CHILDREN

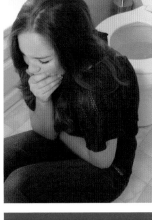

START HERE

VOMITING or "THROWING UP"

▼

- Is your child less than 6 months old?
  or
- Does your child have a fever above 38.5°C (101°F) oral / 39°C (102°F) rectal?
  or
- Do you suspect poisoning?
  or
- Does your child have severe stomach pain?
  or
- Is your child severely ill between vomiting episodes?
  or
- Do you suspect a head injury?
  or
- Is the child diabetic?
  or
- Could the child be pregnant?
  or
- Is there evidence of dehydration? See Ⓐ, page 72, for details.

YES ▶ **GO TO THE HEALTH CENTRE** *or* **HOSPITAL NOW** Ⓗ

NO
▼

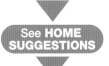
See **HOME SUGGESTIONS**

▼

- Is your child unable to drink fluids and there has been regular hourly vomiting for more than 4 hours?

YES ▶ **GO TO THE HEALTH CENTRE** *or* **HOSPITAL NOW** Ⓗ

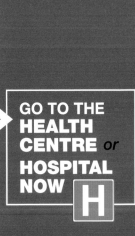

NO
▼

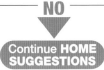
Continue **HOME SUGGESTIONS**

Review this chart from the top every 2 hours.

Vomiting or "the Stomach Flu"
CHILDREN

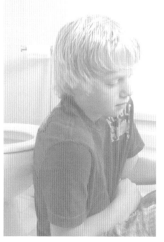

▶ # HOME SUGGESTIONS

(A) Your child may be dehydrated if:

- There are fewer than 4 wet diapers per day or the child has not urinated during the last 8 hours.
- There are no tears when your child cries.
- Your child's mouth is dry or the eyes are sunken.
- Your child is dizzy when they stand.
- Your child is very sleepy and weak.

Important feeding advice for children of all ages

If your child vomits once, give them a 2 hour break from food and fluids to allow the stomach to settle. If they vomit again you must take action to avoid dehydration. Remember the key to caring for a vomiting child is to give small amounts of liquid often. This will usually control the vomiting. Use a medicine dropper, spoon or cup if it helps your child take the fluids. **Give 1 oz every 20 to 30 minutes**.

Many experts would advise that you immediately stop all food and fluids and give oral "rehydration" drinks such as **Gastrolyte** or **Pedialyte** until vomiting stops. We agree that this is ideal to prevent dehydration, but many parents have found that the unpleasant taste of these liquids can make this difficult. You can add unsweetened drink crystals to help improve the taste. Some people make freeze-pops from this mixture for their kids to suck on when ill.

If the vomiting and/or diarrhea is mild we feel it is reasonable to start with clear fluids. This includes water, apple juice, pear juice, flattened ginger ale and popsicles. If there is diarrhea make sure that you dilute the juices with an equal amount of water. If the vomiting continues then we suggest that you switch to the "rehydration" drinks.

A clear fluid diet is only acceptable for 24 hours. After that period you should start using rehydration drinks.

If you are unable to get these fluids into your child and regular vomiting and/or diarrhea continues for more than 4 hours, you should see a doctor. Children with both vomiting and diarrhea must be watched closely for signs of dehydration (see above).

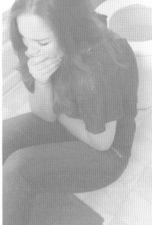

Vomiting or "the Stomach Flu"
CHILDREN

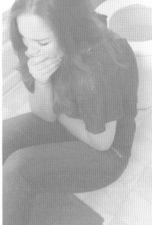

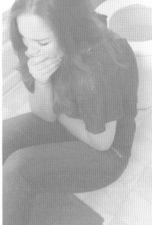

▶ # HOME SUGGESTIONS

How to care for breast-fed babies

1   **Do not stop breast-feeding!** Breast milk is a natural fluid that is easily and rapidly digested. Even if your baby is vomiting, they will absorb some nutrients and fluid before it comes back up.

Nurse for half the length of the time but twice as often as usually. If vomiting continues, reduce the nursing time and feed your child more often. Remember that a sick child becomes tired quickly. For comfort you may have to express some milk and offer a less full breast for feeding. Make sure you read "**Important feeding advice for children of all ages**" on page 72.

2   If your child has a fever please see the **FEVER** section on page 56. If your child has vomited up the medication, you can use suppositories (medication taken rectally) which contains acetaminophen. Ask your pharmacist to help you purchase the right product.

3   Do not give any medication for vomiting to children under 3 years of age. We find that dimenhydrinate (**Gravol**), which is frequently used in older children and adults, is usually unnecessary and we have found it to be unhelpful in younger children.

4   Vomiting which is irregular or infrequent and allows your child to drink some fluids between episodes is not as serious as hourly vomiting. Nevertheless, if irregular or infrequent vomiting should continue for more than 24 hours you should visit your doctor.

5   If your child is normally eating solid food and has not vomited for at least 4 to 6 hours, you are quite safe to reintroduce food. Some experts suggest that you start with bland foods such as rice, cereal, strained bananas, applesauce, bread, crackers, etc. Our advice is to give the give the child healthy food that they like to eat as long as it does not make them sick again. Gradually return to a normal diet within 1 or 2 days.

6   **Frequent handwashing can decrease the spread of infection**.

THE NEXT PAGE HAS ADVICE FOR FORMULA-FED AND OLDER CHILDREN. **FOR A HOMEMADE REHYDRATION DRINK SEE PAGE 113.**

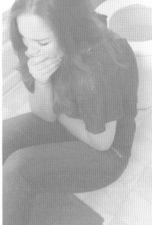

continued next page...

CHILDREN **VOMITING**

Vomiting or "the Stomach Flu"
CHILDREN

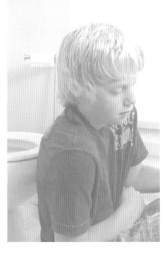

▶ # HOME SUGGESTIONS

How to care for formula-fed babies and older children

1   Make sure you read "Important feeding advice for children of all ages" (page 72).

2   If your child has a fever please see the **FEVER** section on page 56. Suppositories (medication given by rectally) containing acetaminophen can be used when medication taken by mouth won't stay down. Ask your pharmacist to help you purchase the right product.

3   Do not give any medication for vomiting to children under 3 years of age. **Gravol** which is frequently used in older children and adults is usually unnecessary and we have found it to be unhelpful in younger children. A 25 mg dose by mouth or as a rectal suppository can be used in children over age 3.

4   Vomiting which is irregular or infrequent and allows your child to drink some fluids between episodes is not as serious as hourly vomiting. Nevertheless, if irregular or infrequent vomiting should continue for more than 24 hours you should visit your doctor.

5   If your child has not vomited in the last 6 hours, you can restart milk and foods. Many experts suggest that you start with bland foods such as rice, cereal, bread, crackers, potatoes, etc. Our advice is to give the child healthy food that they like as long as it does not make them sick again. Gradually return to a normal diet in 1 to 2 days.

6   **Frequent handwashing can decrease the spread of infection.**

FOR A HOMEMADE REHYDRATION DRINK SEE PAGE 113.

How much fluid should you give your child?

Age	1 year and under		1 - 2 years		over 2 years	
Amount	15 ml *or* 1 tbsp *or* 1/2 oz	▶ every 15 minutes	30 ml *or* 2 tbsp *or* 1 oz	▶ every 15-20 minutes	30-60 ml *or* 2-4 tbsp *or* 1-2 oz	▶ every 15-20 minutes

This is a guide and must be adjusted according to whether fluid losses have been mild or severe. Even if the child is vomiting, continue to give the fluids. The child is always keeping some of the swallowed fluids.

Diarrhea

SUMMARY: Diarrhea is a common problem at any age. A sudden change in diet is a common cause of some short-lived loosening of bowel movements. The rapid onset of frequent, loose bowel movements without bleeding, however, is usually the result of a viral illness or "stomach flu". Mild diarrhea in a child whose intake of fluids and food remains normal is not usually serious and does not require a visit to the doctor. More serious diarrhea requires specific diet planning and close monitoring to make sure that dehydration does not develop. It may take from 7 to 10 days for bowel movements to return to normal. If the diarrhea contains blood you should see a doctor.

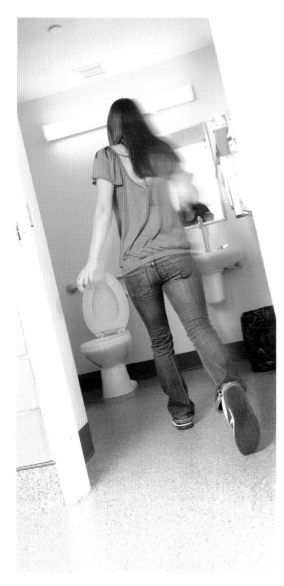

CHILDREN
Possible Symptoms:

▸ loose, frequent, watery bowel movements
▸ cramps
▸ reduced appetite
▸ nausea
▸ vomiting
▸ fever
▸ body aches

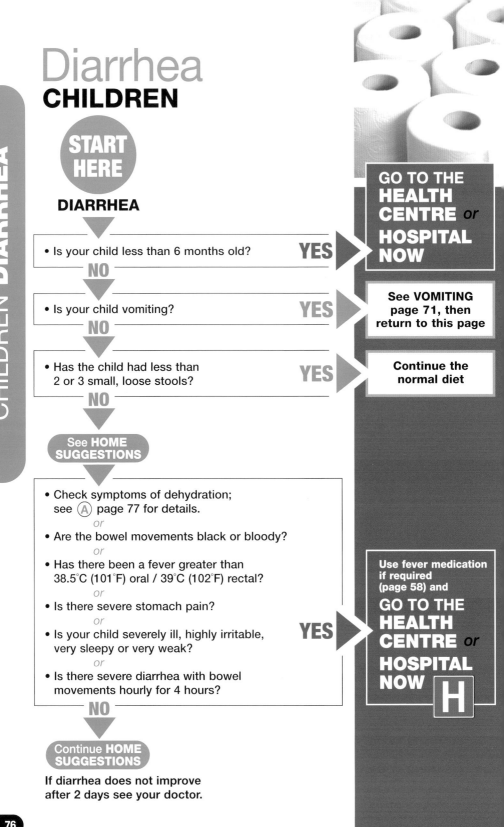

Diarrhea
CHILDREN

START HERE

DIARRHEA

- Is your child less than 6 months old? **YES**

  GO TO THE HEALTH CENTRE *or* **HOSPITAL NOW**

NO

- Is your child vomiting? **YES**

  See VOMITING page 71, then return to this page

NO

- Has the child had less than 2 or 3 small, loose stools? **YES**

  Continue the normal diet

NO

See **HOME SUGGESTIONS**

- Check symptoms of dehydration; see Ⓐ page 77 for details.
  or
- Are the bowel movements black or bloody?
  or
- Has there been a fever greater than 38.5°C (101°F) oral / 39°C (102°F) rectal?
  or
- Is there severe stomach pain?
  or
- Is your child severely ill, highly irritable, very sleepy or very weak?
  or
- Is there severe diarrhea with bowel movements hourly for 4 hours?

YES

Use fever medication if required (page 58) and

GO TO THE HEALTH CENTRE *or* **HOSPITAL NOW** **H**

NO

Continue **HOME SUGGESTIONS**

If diarrhea does not improve after 2 days see your doctor.

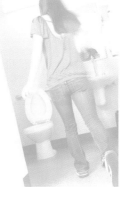

Diarrhea
CHILDREN

▶ # HOME SUGGESTIONS

(A) Your child may be dehydrated if:

- Your child has not urinated for 8 hours.
- There are no tears when your child cries.
- Your child's mouth is dry or the eyes are sunken.
- Your child is dizzy when they stand.
- Your child is very sleepy and weak.

General treatment suggestions for children with diarrhea

If your child has a fever please see the **FEVER** section on page 56.
Your goal in taking care of a child with diarrhea is to make sure they are getting enough to eat and drink so they do not develop dehydration. Otherwise, there is no specific treatment for a viral diarrhea.

Breast or formula-fed children

Don't stop breast-feeding. Whenever possible, maintain the child's intake of solid and liquid food. If the child's stools are very watery or frequent you should give extra fluids between feedings. Sometimes using a spoon or a medicine dropper can help get the child to take the fluid. Many experts would recommend using oral rehydration drinks such as **Gastrolyte** or **Pedialyte** immediately to prevent dehydration. We agree that this is ideal; however, the taste of these products may make it difficult to give these fluids in adequate amounts if the child is not that thirsty. We suggest that water or dilute juice (add equal parts of water and juice) be used for a short period of time for mild and infrequent diarrhea. If vomiting is present or the diarrhea is persistent or severe, we suggest you use the rehydration drinks immediately. If the diarrhea has been present for 5 to 7 days you may want to try and see if a lactose-free or soya-based formula helps to settle the problem. (Pump your breast milk in the meantime so as to preserve the supply.) If you feel that your child is not keeping up with the fluid they are losing, you should see a doctor. The most important thing is to watch for signs of dehydration (see top of the page).

Older children

If milk and a normal solid food diet are tolerated continue to feed normally. You should add additional fluids. Many experts advise the immediate use of oral rehydration drinks such as **Gastrolyte** or **Pedialyte** at this time. We agree that this is ideal and the best way to prevent dehydration. However, some children do not take these drinks well due to their unpleasant taste. You can improve it by adding unsweetened drink crystals.

continued next page...

Diarrhea
CHILDREN

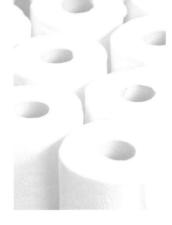

▶ HOME
SUGGESTIONS

1   We feel that for mild and infrequent diarrhea, it is safe to use clear liquids that the child enjoys and will take more easily. Juices should be diluted with an equal amount of water. Soups (chicken soup or consomme), or flattened ginger ale can be used for a short period of time. **Remember that any clear liquid diet is only acceptable for 24 hours**. After that period one should be using rehydration drinks and restarting solids. We recommend your child be given a **minimum of 3 to 6 oz (90 to 180 mls) per hour**. Sometimes using a spoon or a medicine dropper can help get the child to take the fluids.

2   When you are reintroducing food, some experts recommend that you start with bland foods such a rice, cereal, strained bananas, mashed potatoes, bread, etc. Our advice is to give the children healthy food that they like as long as it does not make them sick again. Gradually return to a normal diet in 1 to 2 days.

3   If the diarrhea is prolonged for 5 to 7 days, a lactose-free milk or soya-based formula may be tried for several days to see if the diarrhea slows. If you are unable to get your child to drink well or you feel you are not keeping up with the fluid losses, you should see a doctor.

FOR A HOMEMADE REHYDRATION DRINK SEE PAGE 113.

Constipation

SUMMARY: Constipation has various definitions but if a child cannot pass their stool or if there is obvious pain on passing stool then they need some treatment. Children often need to strain to have a bowel movement. If it is not painful, this is not a concern. Like adults, children may have different bowel habits. A daily bowel movement is not necessary. The hardness of the stool depends on the fibre and water intake as well as the general health of the child. Breast-fed children may not move their bowels more often than once every 7 days. During the first week of life, however, one should expect a daily bowel movement. Any change in diet, especially a change from breast milk to formula or the introduction of cow's milk and solid food may result in a temporary firming up of bowel movements. This change is usually self-correcting. Constipation does not cause fever.

CHILDREN
Possible Symptoms:

▶ infrequent bowel movements

▶ pain with bowel movements

▶ hard and pebble-like stools

▶ unable to move bowels

▶ small tears in the anal canal (fissures)

▶ cramps

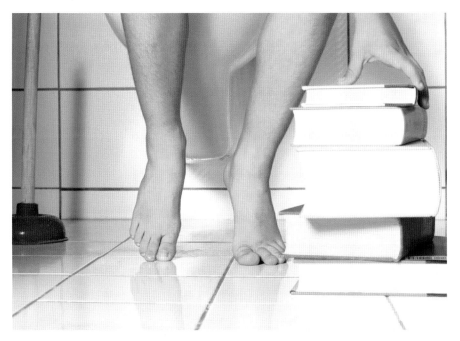

Constipation
CHILDREN

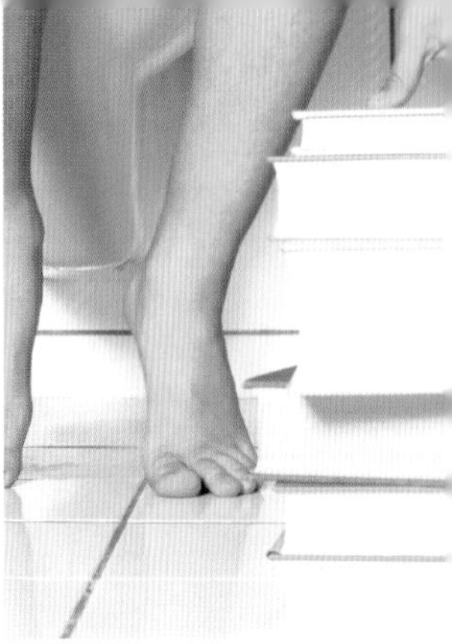

START HERE

POSSIBLE CONSTIPATION

• Are bowel movements soft? — **YES** ▶ **No Treatment Required**

NO

• Is there severe pain or fever?
or
• Does the child look ill? — **YES** ▶ **GO TO THE HEALTH CENTRE** *or* **HOSPITAL NOW** **H**

NO

See **HOME SUGGESTIONS**

• Is the child still constipated? — **YES** ▶ **GO TO THE HEALTH CENTRE** *or* **HOSPITAL**

NO

Continue **HOME SUGGESTIONS**

Constipation
CHILDREN

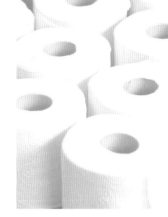

▶ HOME SUGGESTIONS

Children under 6 months of age

Constipation is very rare in this age group so if your child seems constipated, you should visit your doctor.

Children 6 to 12 months of age

1 Encourage your baby to drink more water and fruit juices such as prune, pear, or apple. Give juices at full strength. Do not dilute the juice with water.

2 If your baby is eating solids, increase high fibre foods such as cereals (wheat bran), prunes, beans and pears.

3 Encourage your child to be as active as possible. Exercise can really help this problem and improve your child's overall health.

4 Although mineral oil is sometimes recommended for this age group, we suggest that any **regular** use of laxatives should be given under the supervision of your doctor. Frequently, children need some help to empty the rectum. Using a glycerin suppository or children's enema is a simple and effective treatment. If mineral oil is used, give 1 to 2 tablespoons (15-30 mls) at bedtime. Mineral oil is also available in a mixture of raspberry jelly called **Lansoyl**. An alternative to mineral oil is lactulose. Ask your pharmacist to help purchase any of these treatments for occasional constipation.

Children over 1 year of age

1 Encourage your child to drink more water and fruit juices like prune, pear and apple. Do not dilute juice with water.

2 Increase the fibre in your child's diet with bran, beans, peanut butter, etc. Increasing the quantity of fruits and vegetables your child eats may also help. See **CONSTIPATION: ADULT**, page 114, for more detail.

3 If getting your child to eat foods rich in fibre is difficult, a psyllium fibre substitute may be tried. Try mixing one of these products, such as **Metamucil**, with orange juice or other foods to hide the taste. The smooth variety of **Metamucil** may be easier for a child to take.

4 Don't resort to laxatives, suppositories or enemas too easily. These products are only useful for short-term relief. Constipation requires a long-term solution.

continued next page...

Constipation
CHILDREN

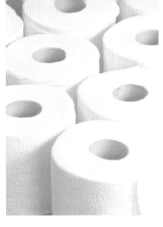

▶ HOME
SUGGESTIONS

5 Laxatives should be used for short-term relief only. See your doctor if laxatives are needed on a regular basis. If your child is having trouble getting the bowel movement started you can use a glycerin suppository or children's enema. If you are going to use a laxative by mouth, we suggest **Milk of Magnesia**. It is given in 1 to 2 tablespoon (15-30 mls) dose once or twice daily. Mineral oil may also be used in a 1 to 2 tablespoon dose at bedtime. An alternative to mineral oil is lactulose. Please ask your pharmacist to help purchase the right product for your child.

6 If your child is toilet trained, try to establish a routine. This means putting the child on the toilet for 5 to 15 minutes at a regular time. Choosing a time which coincides with previous common times for bowel movements or planning these times after meals is a good idea. You will be most successful if you stay away from trying to get your child to use the toilet at stressful times of the day. These would include getting ready for school, just before going out of the house or just prior to bed.

Toilet Training

SUMMARY: Toilet training can be a transition that occurs very easily for some children, while for others it can seem to go on forever. The truth of the matter is that the frustration and stress usually belongs to the parent and not the child. Every developmentally normal child eventually becomes toilet trained even though, at the time, it may not seem that way to a concerned parent.

WHEN IS A CHILD READY?

The most common age to begin toilet training is between 18 and 24 months, but it is not unusual for some children to not be ready until they are three. If your child can signal when their diaper needs to be changed then you can begin to see if they show interest in toilet training. Girls will often master toilet training more quickly and at a younger age than boys.

START HERE

TOILET TRAINING

• Your child can signal you when they need a diaper change? **YES** ▶ **Start Toilet Training** **See next page** ▶HOME SUGGESTIONS

NO

• Age > 3 and you have tried toilet training for longer than 3 to 6 months. **YES** ▶ **See next page** ▶HOME SUGGESTIONS

NO

HAS/IS YOUR CHILD?:
• Recently been ill?
• In a new childcare situation?
• Had trouble passing stool?
• Living in a home that is in the midst of significant change or stress?

YES ▶ **Try Toilet Training again at a later date**

NO

See **HOME SUGGESTIONS**

Toilet Training
CHILDREN

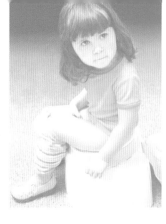

▶ # HOME SUGGESTIONS

1 Begin by buying a potty-chair and leaving it out where the child plays. Let them get on and off it as they please. When they are comfortable with it, you can try letting them sit on it while undressed.

2 Permit the child to watch you use the toilet to take advantage of the natural desire to copy and learn. Let them see stool in the toilet and what happens when they flush.

3 Look for a consistent time of day when your child has a bowel movement and put the child on the potty around this time. Take advantage of the common need to move your bowels after meals. Reading to them or providing some sort of entertainment can increase the child's patience to wait longer while sitting on the potty.

4 Dress the child in loose-fitting clothes that can be quickly and easily removed. Watch for signs that indicate that the child needs to use the potty. Parents can learn to recognize their own child's signals. Changes in facial expression, abruptly stopping play or assuming a certain body position are common signals. You can then quickly remove the necessary clothing and put the child on the potty.

5 Putting stress and pressure on your child may increase the likelihood of failure or delay.

6 Praise and encourage your child for every effort even when it did not end in total success. Be patient. Do not punish a child for failure.

7 If potty training is causing a lot of stress and frustration for you or your child, you should take a break and try it again at a later date.

8 Remember that there is often a pattern of progress and then regression. Progress will follow again, but parents should realize that temporary setbacks are normal. Be patient.

9 Some children may achieve daytime control before night-time or naptime control. You may need to use a diaper or a pull-up while the child sleeps.

Special
Topics for
Teenagers

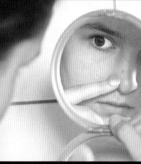

Acne
86

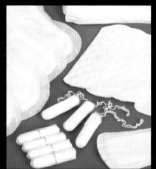

Starting
Menstruation
89

Acne

SUMMARY: As the hormonal changes of adolescence occur, one of the most common and distressing problems to be dealt with is acne. Acne is a skin irritation that occurs on the face and sometimes on the shoulders and chest. The social implications can be more significant than the true threat to health and as a result acne may not get the attention that it deserves. Taking a few steps at home can improve the life and stress of an adolescent.

The rising sex hormone levels of adolescence affect glands in the skin to secrete more oil. This oil, along with skin bacteria, can get trapped in blocked glands and follicles causing the irritation that shows itself as acne.

There are three types of skin problems in acne which often exist in combination in one person:

- Pustules or "whiteheads" form when the skin oil and the bacteria are trapped in a follicle. A small pocket of infection develops and the pus forms the whitehead.

- Blackheads are formed as dead skin plugs the opening of a follicle and with exposure to the air the surface of the plug turns black. They are not typically red or swollen.

- Cystic acne is the most severe form of acne. These tender, inflamed lumps under the skin cannot be popped and you should not try. Cystic acne can form scars and you can increase scarring by picking, squeezing and rubbing your face aggressively. Prescription medication from your doctor is needed for the best result.

There is no medical evidence that diet or poor hygiene causes acne. If you are absolutely convinced that certain foods are aggravating the acne, you can withdraw those foods from your diet.

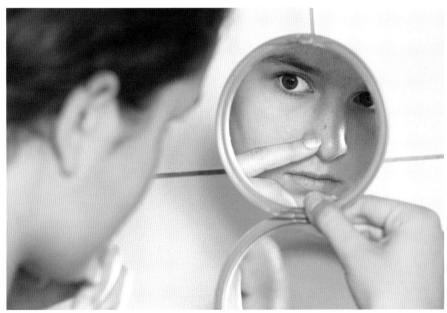

Acne
TEENAGERS

START HERE

YOU HAVE SPOTS ON YOUR FACE, SHOULDERS OR CHEST

- Do you have large (>5mm), tender, red lumps or cysts on your face, shoulders or chest or scars from previous acne (severe acne)?

YES → **See Your Doctor**

NO

- Are you taking medication such as: birth control pills or injections, corticosteroids, hormones, lithium, anti-seizure medication, cyclosporin?

YES → **See Your Doctor**

NO

- Do you have small black dots (blackheads), small red lumps, or white-headed red lesions (whiteheads)(mild to moderate acne)?

YES → **See next page** ► HOME SUGGESTIONS

NO

See your doctor for a diagnosis of your rash

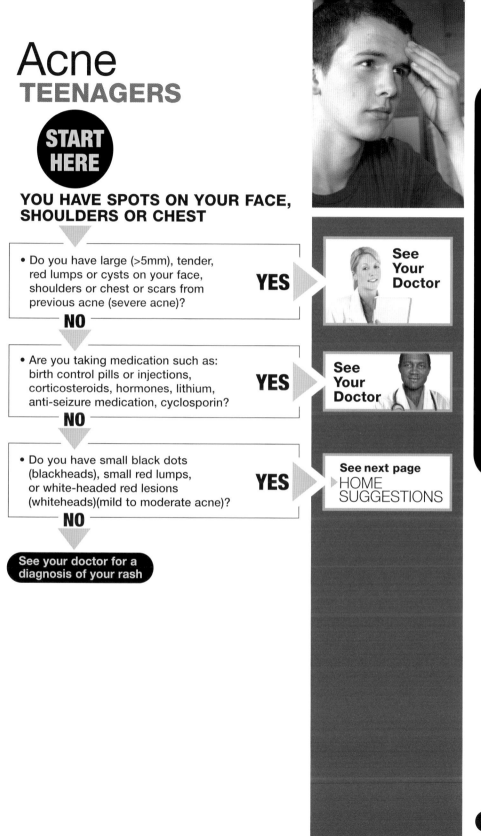

Acne
TEENAGERS

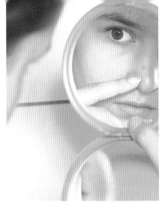

▶ # HOME SUGGESTIONS

Mild or moderate acne can often be controlled at home by following these steps:

1   Avoid picking, popping or aggressively scrubbing any acne.
    Gentle washing with your hands or a warm cloth promotes healing.

2   If you have oily skin you should wash twice a day as this helps decrease the amount of oil and bacteria on the skin.

3   Avoid creams or cosmetics that are oily or greasy. Use only products that are "non-comedogenic." This means that they do not promote pimples (comedones).

4   Sweating can make acne worse, so wash your skin immediately after exercise.

5   If you have oily hair you should wash it daily and try to keep hair off your face.

6   Try to avoid touching or rubbing your face with your hands.

7   Avoid excess exposure to the sun, tanning booths or sun lamps. The sun does not cure acne and some of the medicine you may be taking can make you very sensitive to the sun. Wearing a wide-brimmed hat is a great idea.

8   If you have dry skin and need a moisturizer try a non-comedogenic product such as **Cliniderm Soothing Lotion**.

9   If you need to shave the area, then shave gently with a sharp blade after softening the hair with warm water.

10 Wear cotton under any sports equipment that is rubbing on the areas where you have acne (helmets, chinstraps, shoulder pads).

11 Be patient! It takes time to reduce your acne.

Products that you can use at home to treat mild to moderate acne

1   Benzoyl peroxide (**Clearasil BP Plus**, **Oxy 5**, **Benzagel**). These products are one of the mainstays for treating acne at home.

2   Salicylic acid (**Oxy Daily** cleaning pads, **Clearasil Stayclear**, **Clean and Clear Continuous Control**). These products are used to treat and prevent mild acne and come in lotion, cream, gel or pad form.

3   Acetone and alcohol. (Ask your pharmacist about an astringent available.) These two together work to degrease the skin and have a mild effect against bacteria. They are not as popular due to irritation.

 NOTE: Product lines such as **Clearasil**, **Oxy** and **Clean and Clear** have a multitude of products which contain some of these ingredients, a combination of them, or various other ingredients. It you are not sure what you are selecting, please ask your pharmacist for advice.

Starting
Menstruation

SUMMARY: Adolescence can be a very confusing time of life, and when you add the physical changes that puberty brings, it can become even more distressing. Puberty is a time when hormones change our bodies from those of children to those of adults.

One of the main issues of concern for girls and parents is the timing of the onset of puberty. Age of onset can vary widely from age 8 to 13 years and it can be stressful if someone is at either end of the age range. Usually about two to three years after a girl begins to see development of her breasts, she will begin to have her menstrual cycle. In the few months before her first period, a girl may notice an increased clear vaginal discharge which is due to the hormonal changes occurring in her body. In a short time, she will have her first period or menstrual bleed.

WHAT IS GOING ON? Many girls don't really understand what menstruation is. Approximately once a month, an egg is released from one of the two ovaries and moves into the Fallopian tubes where it may or may not be fertilized by sperm from a male. If it is fertilized, the egg travels into the uterus where it will stay and grow. The lining of the uterus is designed to support and nourish the fertilized egg, but if conception has not occurred, then this lining must be shed before the process starts again with a new egg. The body releases this lining down through the vagina. This process is called "having your period," or menstruation.

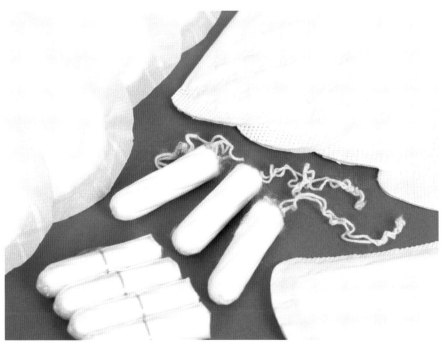

Starting Menstruation

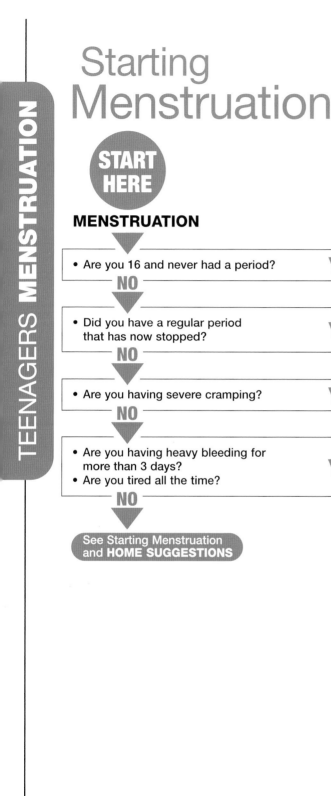

START HERE

MENSTRUATION

- Are you 16 and never had a period? **YES** → **See Your Doctor**

NO

- Did you have a regular period that has now stopped? **YES** → **See Your Doctor**

NO

- Are you having severe cramping? **YES** → **See Your Doctor**

NO

- Are you having heavy bleeding for more than 3 days?
- Are you tired all the time? **YES** → **See Your Doctor**

NO

See Starting Menstruation and **HOME SUGGESTIONS**

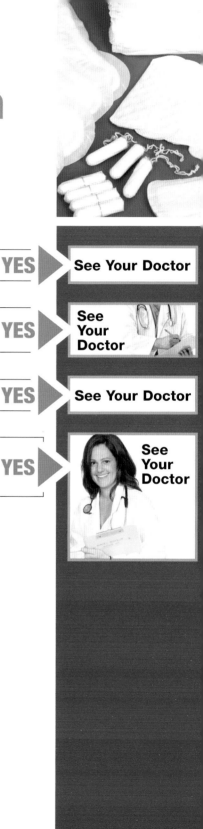

▶ HOME SUGGESTIONS

1 Girls need someone to talk to about starting their period as they often experience a lot of uncertainty. An experienced and open female friend or family member can be greatly appreciated.

2 Some girls may begin to have their period at age 9 and some may not begin until age 15. If a girl is 16 and has not had her period, she should visit her doctor.

3 All girls are born with a genetically determined age at which they will begin their period. What they do or are socially exposed to do not determine timing. Poor nutrition, poor general health and extreme stress can sometimes delay the onset of menstruation. Intense athletic training may also delay the onset of the period.

4 It is normal to have irregular periods in the first year or two. Sometimes a girl may have two periods close together and at other times, she may seem to miss one altogether. This is simply because she is still at an age of hormonal adjustment.

5 Some girls have heavy periods with a lot of bleeding that may last seven days, while other girls pass very little blood and may be done in two or three days. Both of these can be normal.

6 Cramping ranges from minor to so severe that a girl is unable to complete her usual daily schedule. It usually occurs just prior to her period arriving and may last a few days. This does not mean that a health problem exists, but if cramping is unbearable, she should see her doctor. Ibuprofen (**Advil** and others) taken regularly just before and during the period may reduce cramping symptoms.

7 Emotional fluctuations are very common around the time that a girl has her period. This can make a girl seem edgy or irritable while others may be withdrawn, quiet and even feel a little depressed. These changes are common and are known as premenstrual syndrome (PMS). If a girl does not return to her normal self between periods, she should see her doctor.

8 All girls need instruction on how to care for the flow of blood that makes up her period and on how to use tampons and pads. All women have a menstrual cycle for a many years. Don't be afraid to ask for advice from family or friends.

9 If a girl is sexually active and has had a regular period and it does not come at the normal time, this can be a sign that she is pregnant. Pregnancy can occur at any time. Even girls who are not having a period need to use some method of birth control if sexually active.

10 Having sexual activity during menstrual flow is not an effective birth control method.

continued next page...

▶ HOME SUGGESTIONS

While this can be a difficult time of life, menstruation must not be treated like a disease. It must not be treated or referred to as a curse or a penance. Girls should be taught to expect this as a normal part of life that and is a necessary step in becoming a woman. Equally important is the need to encourage girls to continue their usual activities and not let their period interfere with anything they would like to do.

Severe Cramping

For many girls the first few days of their period are marked with severe cramps. These can often be treated successfully by taking regular doses of ibuprofen (see page 58) or a **Midol** product. If ibuprofen upsets your stomach you can try acetaminophen (**Tylenol** and others). Ibuprofen is best taken just before or at the very beginning of your period. This is easier when your periods become more regular because you can predict when cramping will begin. Don't forget that regular exercise throughout the whole cycle can help decrease cramps. A heating pad or taking a warm bath can help. If you have severe cramps that are uncontrollable and regular activities become impossible, a visit to the doctor is wise.

Some women may need to take an iron supplement to prevent anemia caused by heavy bleeding. Heavy bleeding for more than two or three days and bleeding with clots is commonly associated with iron deficiency. If you suffer heavy periods or are feeling increasingly fatigued, you should ask your doctor to check blood (hemoglobin) and iron levels. Taking iron without checking your level can sometimes be dangerous.

The doctor may offer a prescription for a short course of oral contraceptive pills, which are usually very successful in controlling irregular periods, heavy bleeding and severe cramping.

Topics for Adults

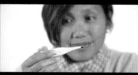
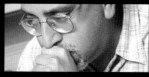
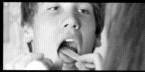
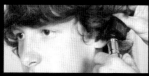
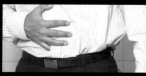
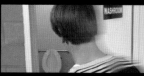
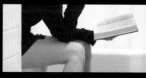
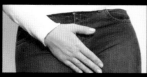
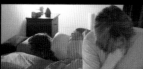
TOPICS FOR ADULTS

Fever
ADULT

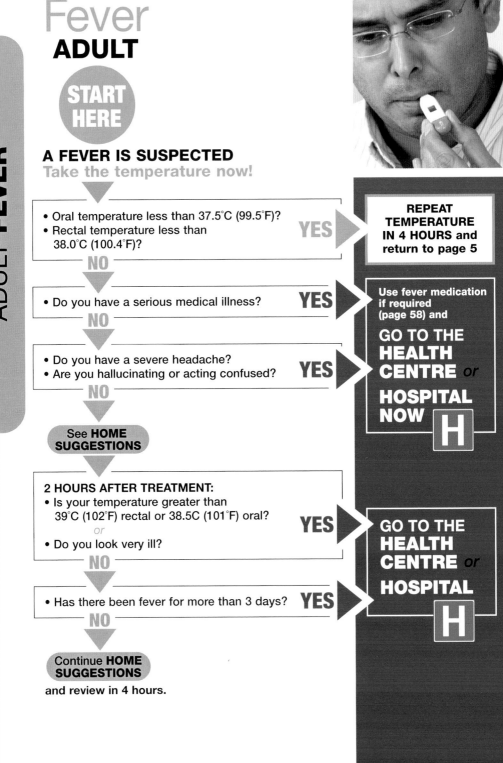

START HERE

A FEVER IS SUSPECTED
Take the temperature now!

- Oral temperature less than 37.5°C (99.5°F)?
- Rectal temperature less than 38.0°C (100.4°F)?

YES → **REPEAT TEMPERATURE IN 4 HOURS and return to page 5**

NO

- Do you have a serious medical illness?

YES →

NO

- Do you have a severe headache?
- Are you hallucinating or acting confused?

YES →

NO

Use fever medication if required (page 58) and

GO TO THE HEALTH CENTRE *or* HOSPITAL NOW **H**

See **HOME SUGGESTIONS**

2 HOURS AFTER TREATMENT:
- Is your temperature greater than 39°C (102°F) rectal or 38.5C (101°F) oral?
  or
- Do you look very ill?

YES →

NO

- Has there been fever for more than 3 days? **YES** →

NO

GO TO THE HEALTH CENTRE *or* HOSPITAL **H**

Continue **HOME SUGGESTIONS**
and review in 4 hours.

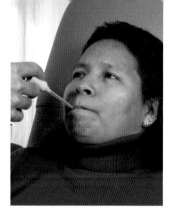

Fever

ADULT

▶ HOME
SUGGESTIONS

1   When the adult patient has a fever, dress lightly and don't cover with blankets.

2   If the patient starts to shiver, dress them warmly until it stops, then dress lightly again.

3   Give acetaminophen (**Tylenol** and others) every 4 hours if the patient is uncomfortable or if the patient's temperature is high (see chart on page 58 for proper dose). Ibuprofen (**Advil**, **Motrin** and others) may be used instead of acetaminophen. Ibuprofen is taken every 6 to 8 hours. Do not use ASA (**Aspirin** and others) in anyone under 20 years of age (see page 178).

4   If the patient vomits the medication given for pain or fever, you can use acetaminophen suppositories (medication given rectally) instead. Ask your pharmacist for help.

5   We suggest that you do not bathe. Bathing may cause shivering which will raise the temperature again.

6   Encourage the patient to drink plenty of liquids. Fluid losses increase with fever.

7   Take the temperature at least every 4 hours and certainly if the fever is worse.

8   If the patient complains of a sore throat, cough, earache or other problems, please review these topics as well.

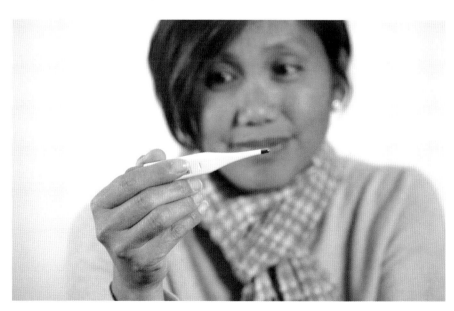

Cough & Cold
and "the Flu"

SUMMARY: Colds are caused by viruses and do not have a specific treatment at this time. **Taking an antibiotic will not cure your cold.** The flowchart will help you decide if you need to see a doctor. During the course of a year adults may get several colds which may vary in the amount of discomfort they cause. Some may go almost unnoticed, while others cause severe symptoms. **The very old, and those with lung disease, diabetes, heart disease or other chronic illnesses may require a visit to the doctor sooner.** Normally, a cold will get better in 7 to 14 days whether you see a doctor or not. Some symptoms may last longer. A dry cough which may develop during a cold may last 2 to 3 weeks.

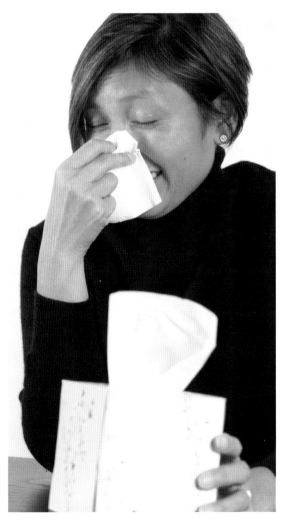

ADULT
Possible Symptoms:

▸ cough
▸ sore throat
▸ body and joint aches
▸ swollen glands in the neck
▸ mild headache
▸ watery eyes
▸ fever
▸ fatigue

Cough & Cold
and "the Flu"
ADULT

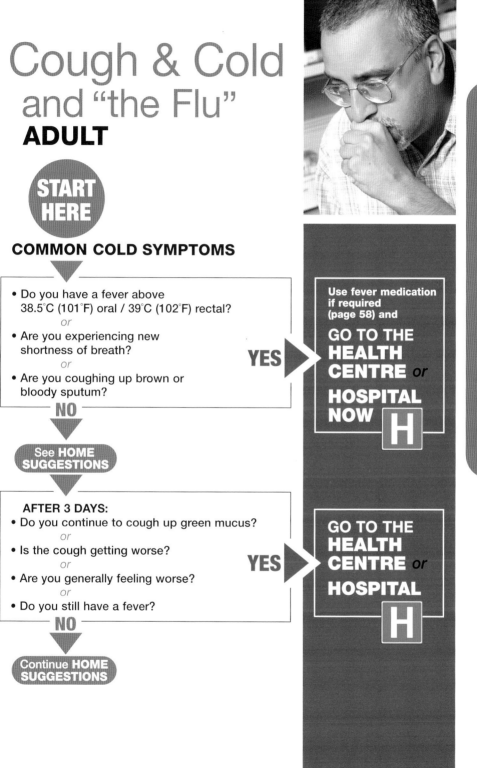

START HERE

COMMON COLD SYMPTOMS

▼

- Do you have a fever above 38.5°C (101°F) oral / 39°C (102°F) rectal?
  or
- Are you experiencing new shortness of breath?
  or
- Are you coughing up brown or bloody sputum?

NO ▼

YES ▶

Use fever medication if required (page 58) and

GO TO THE HEALTH CENTRE *or* **HOSPITAL NOW** **H**

See **HOME SUGGESTIONS**

▼

AFTER 3 DAYS:
- Do you continue to cough up green mucus?
  or
- Is the cough getting worse?
  or
- Are you generally feeling worse?
  or
- Do you still have a fever?

NO ▼

YES ▶

GO TO THE HEALTH CENTRE *or* **HOSPITAL** **H**

Continue **HOME SUGGESTIONS**

Cough & Cold
and "the Flu"
ADULT

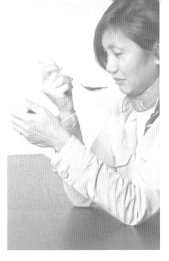

▶ HOME
SUGGESTIONS

Remember, there is no cure for the common cold.
Antibiotics will not shorten the cold or cure it.
You can, however, help yourself to feel better by following these suggestions:

1 Rest and drink plenty of fluids to replace what you lose from a runny nose, cough and fever.

2 Use acetaminophen (**Tylenol** and others), ASA (**Aspirin** and others) or Ibuprofen (**Advil**, **Motrin** or others) for the fever, aches and pains. We do not recommend ASA for those under 20 years of age (see page 178 for further advice). See page 58 for acetaminophen dosage.

3 Humidified air may help the cold symptoms. Use a cool mist humidifier. We suggest you avoid ultrasonic humidifiers and hot mist humidifiers.

4 Standing in a hot shower may help a congested head. Do this as often as you find helpful.

5 Drink hot liquids. These can help a congested nose, and loosen a cough. Chicken soup and hot lemon drinks are good suggestions.

6 You can try a decongestant for the head congestion and runny nose. Combination medications containing a decongestant and an antihistamine, such as **Dimetapp**, may improve sleep. Ask your pharmacist for assistance. See page 176. Those with severe heart disease, poorly controlled blood pressure, angina, or asthma should not take decongestant medications.

7 Cough syrups with "DM" (dextromethorphan) may be used to ease a dry cough. You should not suppress all coughing. A loose or congested cough is helping you clear mucus from the air passages. A cough medicine may be used if you are not sleeping well or you are finding it difficult to work because of the cough. "DM" containing products may make asthma worse. Use them with caution.

8 Coughs and sneezes spread infection. We recommend covering your mouth and nose, but most importantly, remember to wash your hands after you cough or you can spread the infection by touching people. Handwashing is very important in preventing the spread of your cold to other family members and co-workers.

9 Do not smoke or expose yourself to second-hand smoke.

10 See **SORE THROAT** page 99 and **FEVER** page 94 if necessary.

Sore Throat

SUMMARY: Most sore throats are part of a viral infection also causing a cough or cold. These viral infections cannot be cured with antibiotics. If you develop severe pain, high fever, a rash, or have a lot of difficulty swallowing, you should see a doctor. In most cases your sore throat will get better in 1 week or less. This flowchart will help you decide if you should see your doctor about your sore throat. Because antibiotics do not help the pain immediately, night-time visits to the emergency department for antibiotics are not usually necessary. Use the **HOME SUGGESTIONS** for some early relief of the pain.

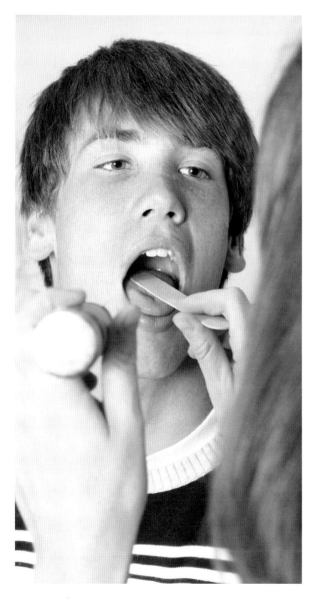

ADULT
Possible Symptoms:

▸ sore throat
▸ pain on swallowing
▸ fever
▸ swollen neck glands
▸ hoarse voice or laryngitis
▸ red throat or pus on tonsils

Sore Throat
ADULT

START HERE

SORE THROAT
(If accompanied by other cold symptoms see also COUGH AND COLD)

- Do you have a temperature greater than 38.5°C (101°F) oral / 39°C (102°F) rectal?
  or
- Are you having a lot of difficulty with swallowing or breathing?
  or
- Do you have a new skin rash?
  or
- Do you have a severe sore throat alone without the symptoms of a runny nose, cough or cold?

YES ▶ Use fever medication if required (page 58) and **GO TO THE HEALTH CENTRE** or **HOSPITAL NOW** **H**

NO

See **HOME SUGGESTIONS**

- Are you swallowing easier with home therapy? **NO** ▶ **GO TO THE HEALTH CENTRE** or **HOSPITAL**

YES

Continue **HOME SUGGESTIONS**

- Is the sore throat still severe or getting worse after 2 or 3 days? **YES** ▶ **GO TO THE HEALTH CENTRE** or **HOSPITAL**

NO

Review this chart from the top in 24 hours.

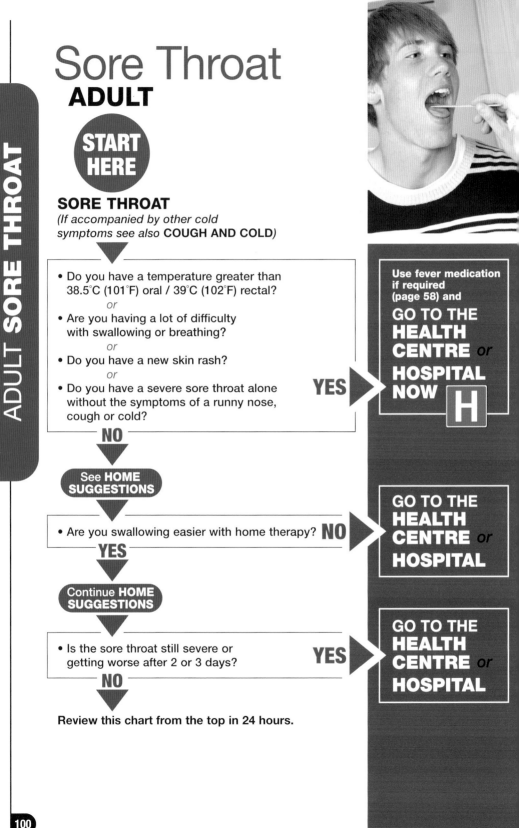

Sore Throat
ADULT

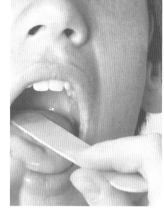

▶ HOME SUGGESTIONS

1 Get plenty of rest and drink extra fluids.

2 Use acetaminophen (**Tylenol** and others), ASA (**Aspirin** and others) or ibuprofen (**Advil**, **Motrin** and others) for pain and fever. We do not recommend ASA for those under 20 years of age (see page 178 for further advice). See page 58 for acetaminophen dosage.

3 You may find that gargles or anesthetic ("numbing or freezing") medications may reduce the pain and help you to eat. Using a warm salt water gargle or double strength tea may also give some relief. Combining 8 oz of warm water with 1 teaspoon of salt and 1 or 2 tablespoons of corn syrup or honey makes a soothing gargle. Products such as **Chloraseptic** which contain 0.5% phenol and flavouring may also be used with good results.

4 Suck on a lozenge or hard candy to help soothe your throat.

5 A cool mist humidifier is helpful. We suggest that you avoid ultrasonic and hot mist humidifiers.

6 Apply warm compresses to the sore neck glands for 30 minutes 4 to 6 times daily.

7 You may find that soft foods, soups and liquids are easier to swallow for the first 2 to 3 days.

8 If you have a hoarse voice (laryngitis), try to rest your voice. If your hoarse voice does not improve within 2 to 3 weeks you should see your doctor.

 "Beware of the lone sore throat. A severe sore throat without, cough, runny nose or chest congestion should be seen by a doctor."

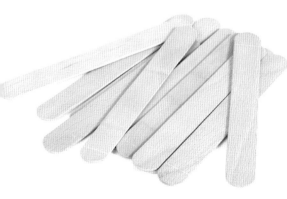

Earache

SUMMARY: Ear infections can occur in the ear canal, or behind the ear drum. Ear canal infections may develop after a day of swimming or water play (sometimes called "swimmer's ear"). The ear canal may become irritated and infected more often if you use cotton swabs to "clean" the ear canal.
Infections behind the ear drum, called "middle ear" infections may develop during viral infections such as the cold or flu. During a cold there can be swelling and congestion which blocks the normal drainage through the Eustachian tube.
HOME SUGGESTIONS may help in easing the discomforts of an ear infection, and help you decide when you should visit your doctor.

ADULT
Possible Symptoms:

- pain in or around the ear
- an itchy ear
- poor hearing
- discharge from the ear
- fever
- sore glands around the ear or in neck
- pain when the ear is tugged

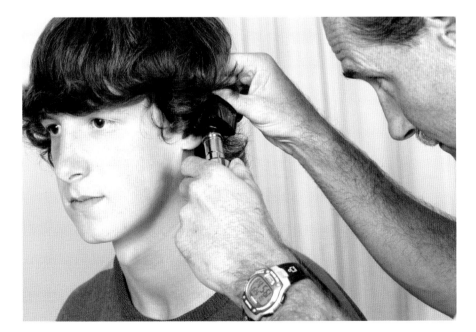

Earache
ADULT

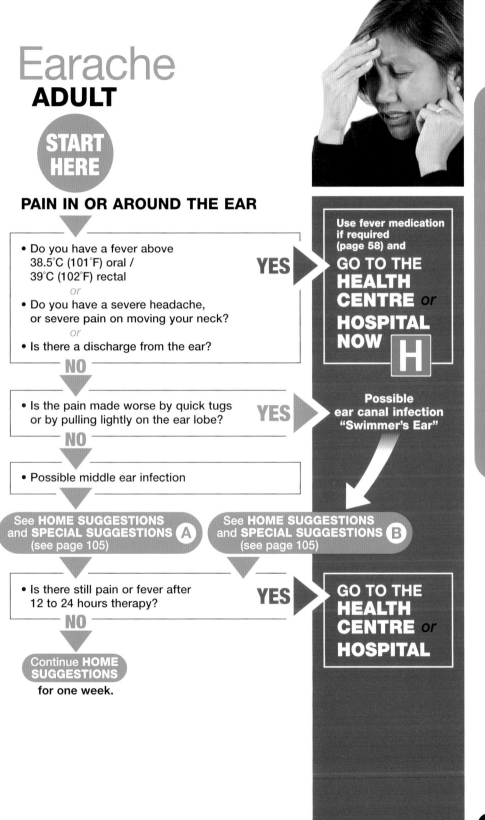

START HERE

PAIN IN OR AROUND THE EAR

- Do you have a fever above 38.5°C (101°F) oral / 39°C (102°F) rectal
  or
- Do you have a severe headache, or severe pain on moving your neck?
  or
- Is there a discharge from the ear?

YES ➤ Use fever medication if required (page 58) and

GO TO THE HEALTH CENTRE *or* **HOSPITAL NOW** **H**

NO

- Is the pain made worse by quick tugs or by pulling lightly on the ear lobe?

YES ➤ **Possible ear canal infection "Swimmer's Ear"**

NO

- Possible middle ear infection

See **HOME SUGGESTIONS** and **SPECIAL SUGGESTIONS** **A** (see page 105)

See **HOME SUGGESTIONS** and **SPECIAL SUGGESTIONS** **B** (see page 105)

- Is there still pain or fever after 12 to 24 hours therapy?

YES ➤ **GO TO THE HEALTH CENTRE** *or* **HOSPITAL**

NO

Continue **HOME SUGGESTIONS** for one week.

Earache
ADULT

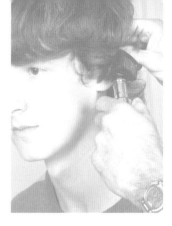

▶ HOME SUGGESTIONS

If you have a fever, please see the **FEVER** section on page 94.

1 Most people are very anxious to control the pain caused by middle ear infections. Use acetaminophen (**Tylenol** and others), ASA (**Aspirin** and others) or ibuprofen (**Advil**, **Motrin** and others). See page 178 for pain medication use. See page 58 for acetaminophen dosage. If there is no improvement in the pain or condition within 24 to 36 hours, it may be necessary to take a course of antibiotics. Antibiotics do not relieve pain immediately. We recommend treating yourself with pain medication early and seeking advice about antibiotics during the light of day.

2 Put a warm cloth on the ear for 20 minutes several times daily. This will often help relieve pain.

3 Warm oil drops in the ear canal may give some relief from pain—try **Auralgan** drops or mineral oil, cooking oil or olive oil. Touch your skin with the oil to test how hot it is before putting it in your ear canal.

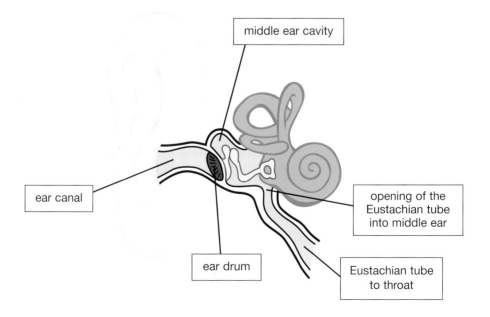

middle ear cavity

ear canal

opening of the Eustachian tube into middle ear

ear drum

Eustachian tube to throat

Earache
ADULT

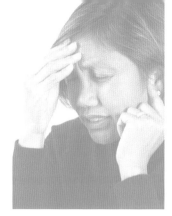

▶ HOME SUGGESTIONS

SPECIAL SUGGESTIONS (A)
For middle ear infections:

1 You can sometimes help relieve discomfort by treating the early symptoms of nasal congestion and ear fullness with decongestants. These agents may help middle ear draining. See page 176 for further information about decongestants. People with severe heart disease, poorly controlled high blood pressure or severe asthma should not use decongestant medications.

2 Try to "pop" your ears by blowing gently with your mouth closed and your nose pinched. Do this several times daily.

SPECIAL SUGGESTIONS (B)
For ear canal infections ("Swimmer's Ear"):

1 Do not get water in your ear for 7 days, if possible. If you do, shake your head to remove it. You can also use a blow dryer on low setting, held 6 to 12 inches from the ear, to dry the ear canal. A few drops of a drying agent will help the ear dry faster. **Buro-sol** or a mixture of 1 tablespoon vinegar and 1 tablespoon of warm water make good drying agents.

2 This is an infection which may respond to non-prescription antibiotic drops (**Polysporin**). Use 2 drops 4 times daily.

3 **DO NOT TRY TO CLEAN OUT THE EAR WITH A COTTON SWAB.** This may increase your risk of ear infections.

4 You may want to prevent another ear canal infection. Placing a couple of drops of an antibiotic solution (**Polysporin**) in the ear after a day of swimming or putting a couple of drops of cooking oil, olive oil or mineral oil in the ear canal before swimming may prevent repeat infections. Ear plugs designed to prevent water from getting in the ear canal may also be helpful. You should not use hard plastic ear plugs.

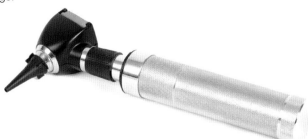

Vomiting or "the Stomach Flu"

SUMMARY: The most common cause of nausea and vomiting (throwing up) is a viral infection usually called "the stomach flu". Most people recover from this illness within 1 or 2 days. Short-lived nausea and vomiting may also occur after eating a bacterial toxin in food; this is commonly called food poisoning.
No specific treatment exists for viral infections or food poisoning of this type. Following our **HOME SUGGESTIONS** will help you relieve the discomfort of this illness. Sometimes nausea and/or vomiting may be caused by medication. If you have started a new prescription medication see your doctor. Women should check to see if they are pregnant.

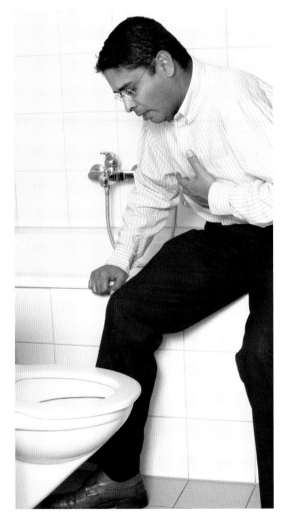

ADULT
Possible Symptoms:

▶ nausea (upset stomach)

▶ vomiting ("throwing up")

And some or all of the following:

▶ diarrhea

▶ fever

▶ headache

▶ dehydration

Vomiting or "the Stomach Flu"
ADULT

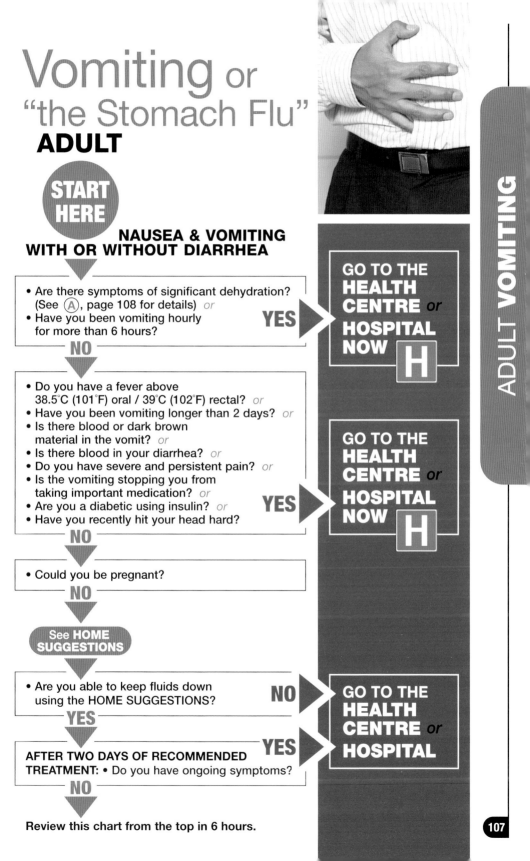

START HERE

NAUSEA & VOMITING WITH OR WITHOUT DIARRHEA

- Are there symptoms of significant dehydration? (See Ⓐ, page 108 for details) *or*
- Have you been vomiting hourly for more than 6 hours?

YES → GO TO THE **HEALTH CENTRE** *or* **HOSPITAL NOW** Ⓗ

NO

- Do you have a fever above 38.5°C (101°F) oral / 39°C (102°F) rectal? *or*
- Have you been vomiting longer than 2 days? *or*
- Is there blood or dark brown material in the vomit? *or*
- Is there blood in your diarrhea? *or*
- Do you have severe and persistent pain? *or*
- Is the vomiting stopping you from taking important medication? *or*
- Are you a diabetic using insulin? *or*
- Have you recently hit your head hard?

YES → GO TO THE **HEALTH CENTRE** *or* **HOSPITAL NOW** Ⓗ

NO

- Could you be pregnant?

NO

See **HOME SUGGESTIONS**

- Are you able to keep fluids down using the HOME SUGGESTIONS?

NO → GO TO THE **HEALTH CENTRE** *or* **HOSPITAL**

YES

AFTER TWO DAYS OF RECOMMENDED TREATMENT: • Do you have ongoing symptoms?

YES → GO TO THE **HEALTH CENTRE** *or* **HOSPITAL**

NO

Review this chart from the top in 6 hours.

Vomiting or "the Stomach Flu"
ADULT

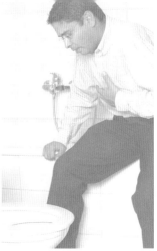

▶ # HOME SUGGESTIONS

Ⓐ Symptoms of dehydration:

- You have not urinated for 8 to 10 hours.
- You do not sweat when you are hot.
- You have a very dry mouth and an intense thirst.
- You feel dizzy when you stand up.
- Confusion, fever, general weakness.

Suggestions for treating nausea and vomiting

1 Most nausea and vomiting will pass in less than 12 hours. If you rest and avoid taking anything but sips of water by mouth for a few hours you may not need any other treatment. Severe repeated vomiting or vomiting of blood will require an immediate visit to your doctor or hospital.

2 After 8 hours it is important to begin to drink some fluid to avoid dehydration. Diarrhea causes an increase in the loss of fluid and you may need to take some medicine to help keep fluids down. See #4 on next page for details. Using clear fluids to start is best. Water, boullion, fruit drinks (avoiding apple or citrus fruits if diarrhea is present), flat ginger ale or oral "rehydration" drinks, such as **Gastrolyte**, are all acceptable. Small amounts of fluid will usually stay down more easily than large amounts. Start with 1 oz, 30 mls or 2 tablespoons every 10 minutes. A clear fluids diet is only acceptable for 24 hours. After that period you should be using rehydration drinks.

3 Avoid milk products during the first 24 hours of your illness. If diarrhea seems to start or increase when you drink milk, then avoid milk products until bowel movements have returned to normal. If your vomiting has stopped, then you can slowly start to introduce healthy food. Some experts recommend starting with bland food such as toast, rice, potatoes, etc. and avoiding spicy foods and meats for a day or two. We suggest that you reintroduce food that you like in small quantities to start, but return to a full diet as your symptoms improve in 2 to 3 days.

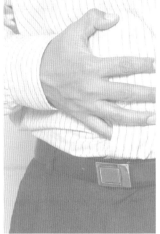

Vomiting or "the Stomach Flu"
ADULT

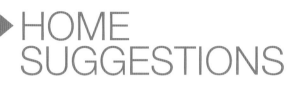

▶ # HOME SUGGESTIONS

4   You can use dimenhydrinate (**Gravol**), a non-prescription medicine to settle nausea. Ask your pharmacist for advice about this medicine. **Gravol** is safe during pregnancy. Dimenhydrinate is available in regular pills, chewable tablets and suppositories (medication given rectally). Adults will require 50 mg every 3 to 4 hours. **Gravol** is a form of antihistamine and may cause sleepiness. Do not drive while taking **Gravol**.

5   Severe diarrhea can sometimes be controlled by using loperimide (**Imodium**). This medicine should be used only for a few days. Loperimide is especially valuable if one must go out of the home while ill. Ask your pharmacist for this medication and instructions. Do not take loperimide if you have a high fever (39°C or 102°F taken orally) or if your stool contains blood.

6   If you are on regular medication for other health problems then you should try to take your medicine with sips of water. If you have missed 2 or more doses then you should seek medical advice.

7   People with diabetes requiring insulin may become very ill if they develop diarrhea or vomiting. Please go to the hospital early.

FOR A HOMEMADE REHYDRATION DRINK SEE PAGE 113.

Diarrhea

SUMMARY: A short episode of non-bloody, loose or watery bowel movements is common for all age groups. The most common cause is a viral infection. Bacterial toxins ("food poisoning") can also cause diarrhea. Both will usually resolve on their own. The infection may be passed between family members, so wash your hands carefully to prevent the spread of the condition. Occasionally a change in diet or a new medication may cause some loose stool. If this does not improve by itself within a few days you should see your doctor. Since the diarrhea will usually resolve by itself, your self-care involves avoiding dehydration and watching for signs of more serious problems as outlined in the flowchart.

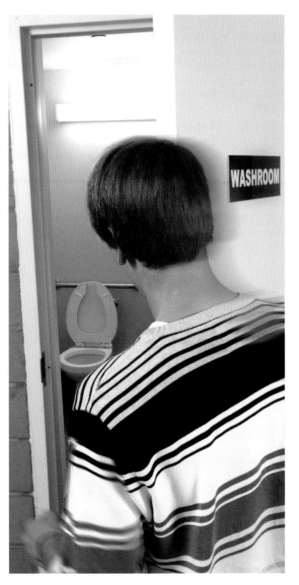

ADULT

Possible Symptoms:

▸ loose, frequent, watery bowel movements

▸ cramps

▸ gas

▸ pain around the anus

▸ nausea and vomiting

▸ bloating

▸ headache

▸ fever

Diarrhea
ADULT

START HERE

DIARRHEA

• Do you have nausea or vomiting? **YES** → Go to **VOMITING** page 106, then return to this page

NO

• Is there blood in the stool? (Not just on the toilet paper) *or*
• Have you a fever above 38.5°C (101°F) oral / 39°C (102°F) rectal? *or*
• Do you have severe abdominal pain? *or*
• Are there signs of dehydration? (See Ⓐ, page 108)

YES → Use fever medication if required (page 58), **GO TO THE HEALTH CENTRE or HOSPITAL NOW** **H**

NO

• Have you been taking a new medicine? (especially antibiotics)

YES → If this is a prescription medicine you should call your doctor. If this is a non-prescription medicine you should stop it and see if the diarrhea stops.

NO

See **HOME SUGGESTIONS**

• Have the symptoms lasted for more than 7 days without improvement?

YES → **GO TO THE HEALTH CENTRE or HOSPITAL**

NO

Continue **HOME SUGGESTIONS**

If diarrhea does not improve after two days see your doctor.

Diarrhea
ADULT

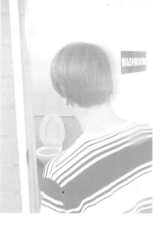

▶ HOME
SUGGESTIONS

Ⓐ Symptoms of dehydration:

- You have not urinated for 8 to 10 hours.
- You do not sweat when you are hot.
- You have a very dry mouth and an intense thirst.
- You feel dizzy when you stand up.
- Confusion, fever, general weakness.

1 It is a good idea to reduce the amount of fibre, caffeine, spicy food and alcohol in your diet for a few days until your condition improves. Otherwise, it is perfectly all right to eat your normal diet, so long as you feel well doing so. Don't eat things that seem to make the diarrhea worse, but there is no diet advice that will work for all people. It is important to drink some extra fluids. If solid food causes more diarrhea, take more fluids instead.

2 While you have diarrhea don't eat candy or artificially sweetened foods. Drink fewer citrus juices and apple juice; these can make the diarrhea worse. Grape and pineapple juices often satisfy a taste for a fruit juice without causing more trouble. Milk products should be avoided until your condition improves. If there is an increase in the diarrhea when you start eating milk products again, then stop until the diarrhea has completely resolved.

3 A new prescription medication can have an effect on your bowels. Antibiotics are often the cause of diarrhea. Try to avoid products that contain magnesium (this includes many antacids). If you have been using a new non-prescription or over-the-counter product of any kind consider stopping it to see if this helps. Frequently a change in your stools caused by a medication only lasts a short time and will correct itself within a few days even if the medication is continued. If the diarrhea is not severe and appears to be as a result of a new medication, you might consider watching the symptom for a few days before seeing your doctor.

4 You can avoid becoming dehydrated by drinking lots of liquids such as water, fruit juices (grape or pineapple) or clear soup. Although they don't taste very good, oral "rehydration" drinks, such as **Pedialyte** or **Gastrolyte**, are very helpful in supplying the fluid and salts you need. These products can be mixed with sugarfree **Kool-Aid** to improve their taste. In general, we suggest you start by drinking fluids that you like. If diarrhea becomes severe or prolonged, we advise a switch to "rehydration" drinks.

▶ HOME
SUGGESTIONS

5 Loperimide (**Imodium**) is a non-prescription or over-the-counter medication that can slow diarrhea. If you need to leave the house this can be useful. However, it will not speed your recovery. It should not be used if you see blood in the stool or if you have high fever (39°C rectal or 38.5C oral), severe pain, nausea or vomiting.

Other medicines used for diarrhea include kaolin and pectin (**Kaopectate** and others), **Wild Strawberry** and bismuth salts, such as **Peptobismol**. Serious diarrhea will not respond to these products. **Peptobismol** should not be given to anyone under 20 years of age when they have a viral illness. See page 178 for an explanation.

6 Review other topics, such as **FEVER** or **VOMITING** if necessary.

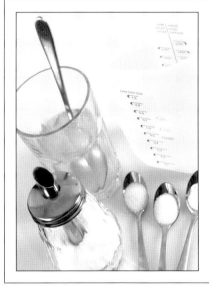

Homemade Rehydration Drink

- 1 LITRE OF WATER
- 1/2 TEASPOON BAKING SODA
- 1/2 TEASPOON SALT
- 3-4 TABLESPOONS SUGAR
- IF AVAILABLE 1/4 TABLESPOON OF "LITE SALT"

ADD UNSWEETENED DRINK CRYSTALS FOR FLAVOURING

Constipation

SUMMARY: Different people have different bowel movement patterns. These patterns vary depending on how much exercise you get, your lifestyle and your overall general health.

Bowel activity is most influenced by how much insoluble fibre (such as wheat bran) you eat and fluids you drink. Some people will move their bowels 3 times daily, while other people may only move their bowels 3 times weekly. There is no rule that everyone should move their bowels every day. Constipation usually means there has been a change to bowel movements that occur less often and may be harder or more difficult to pass.

Constipation can be caused by some of the medication that people take. Some medications which commonly cause constipation include narcotics (codeine, morphine, etc.), aluminum containing antacids and certain high blood pressure medications.

North Americans generally eat low fibre diets. The fibre in your diet comes from the parts of plants that you cannot break down in your digestive system. There are different types of fibre. Wheat bran and coarse grains are the most effective in regulating bowel activity. Please see the **HOME SUGGESTIONS** for further advice about fibre.

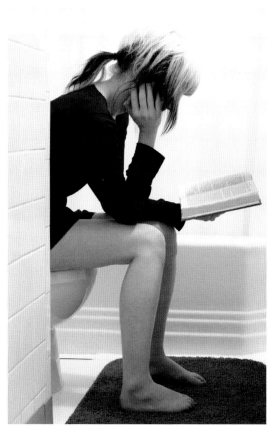

ADULT
Possible Symptoms:

▶ infrequent bowel movements
▶ pain with bowel movements
▶ hard and pebble-like stools
▶ unable to move bowels
▶ small tears in the anal canal (fissures)
▶ cramps

Constipation
ADULT

START HERE

CONSTIPATION
▼

- Are you using laxatives or stool softeners more than twice a week?
  or
- Have you noticed any bleeding?
  or
- Do you have ongoing pain?
  or
- Are you losing weight?

YES ▶ **GO TO THE HEALTH CENTRE** *or* **HOSPITAL**

NO
▼

- Has there been recent non-prescription or prescription medication use?

YES ▶ **Stop taking the non-prescription medication if possible. Continue the prescription medication, and See next page** ▶ HOME SUGGESTIONS

NO
▼

See **HOME SUGGESTIONS**
▼

- After 2 weeks of HOME SUGGESTIONS, are you still constipated?

YES ▶ **GO TO THE HEALTH CENTRE** *or* **HOSPITAL**

NO
▼

Continue **HOME SUGGESTIONS**

Constipation

ADULT

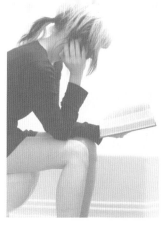

▶ HOME SUGGESTIONS

1   You can use mild laxatives such as **Milk of Magnesia** at a dose of 2 tablespoons (30cc) once or twice daily. You should be careful when you use other laxatives. These usually contain a senna plant product (**Exlax**, **Correctol**, **Sennakot**, many herbal laxatives). These ingredients are harsh and can cause other bowel problems when used regularly. Just because a product has a mild sounding name, or a nicely coloured box, does not mean it contains mild ingredients. Often people only need help starting the bowels to move. This can be helped with a glycerin suppository, or **Fleet** enema. Rarely a more potent suppository is needed. **Dulcolax** suppositories can be used no more than once a week without a doctor's advice.

2   Stool softeners such as docusate sodium or docusate calcium (**Colace**, **Surfak**) may help short-term constipation that is caused by medication, pregnancy, a new illness, a change of diet or a change in life situation.

3   To improve bowel activity in the long run, most people need to add more fibre to their daily diet. The best choice is wheat bran. The secret is to add the fibre in a slow but steady fashion.

    Fibre is not a laxative. It may improve mild diarrhea as much as it may improve constipation. Start with one heaping tablespoon daily of raw wheat bran or 1/4 cup of an all bran cereal (**All Bran**, **Bran Buds** and others). Wait at least one week between increases in your daily intake. If you tolerate the fibre increases you can add 1 tablespoon of raw bran or 1/4 cup of all bran cereal to your daily dose each week. Aim for 2 to 6 tablespoons of raw bran or 1/2 to 1 cup of all bran cereal every day. Psyllium containing products (**Metamucil**, **Prodiem Plain** and others) may also be used as fibre supplements. Remember that the slow but progressive increase in fibre will reduce the development of new symptoms or unwanted side-effects.

    Adding more fibre to your diet by eating more beans, fruits and raw vegetables will also improve your general health, and will make it easier to move your bowels. Be aware that not all plants contain the same kinds of fibre and may not result in the same improvement. Some will have no effect such as oat bran; others may increase gas, such as beans. Eating a higher fibre diet with reduced fat is a good idea for all people. Increasing evidence suggests that there is a reduced risk for cancer and heart disease in people who eat a higher fibre diet.

Constipation
ADULT

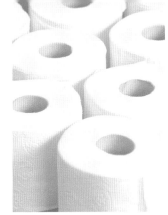

▶ # HOME SUGGESTIONS

4 The Irritable Bowel Syndrome is a condition where a person's bowel activity is constantly changing. People with this condition often have normal or constipated bowel movements, followed by diarrhea which is accompanied by cramping pain. The symptoms of this condition may respond to the fibre advice above but if there are other symptoms that do not respond you should see your doctor. Symptoms of weight loss, rectal bleeding or severe diarrhea should be reported to your doctor.

5 Drinking more water by itself will not make passing stools easier; however, if you are eating more fibre, then you should drink an extra one or two glasses of water per day. The increased fibre will hold the water in the stool and soften it.

6 Passing hard stool may cause you to develop hemorrhoids, or cause some bleeding from the anus. This bleeding is usually bright red and on the surface of the stool, on the paper only, or drips into the toilet. If bleeding occurs frequently, or does not improve with a softening of the stool, you should see your doctor.

Problems with Urination: MEN

SUMMARY: As men age, there is a tendency for the prostate gland to enlarge and create a restriction on the flow of urine out of the bladder. This restriction may result in a slow reduction in the power of the stream and may make it harder to completely empty the bladder. Poor bladder emptying can increase the chance of infection in the bladder. The prostate may also become infected which can cause the prostate to swell and reduce the flow even more. This prostate enlargement is very common and is not directly related to the development of prostate cancer, but if you have experienced a change in your urinary function, it is wise to have your prostate examined by your doctor.

Possible Symptoms:

▸ reduced urine flow

▸ inability to relieve the sense of a full bladder

▸ burning pain in the penis

▸ frequent urination of small quantities

▸ urination increasingly interrupting sleep

▸ incontinence of urine

▸HOME SUGGESTIONS

1   It is not always necessary to use prescription medications for this symptom. Reducing the amount of urine that one makes in the evening may reduce the need to urinate through the night. Reducing or eliminating the intake of fluid for three to four hours before bedtime may help you sleep through the night.

2   Many men improve urine flow by taking saw palmetto (Serenoa repens). This herbal product is available without a prescription and works by shrinking the size of the prostate. Saw palmetto may take up to three months to work, and if there is no improvement in three months, stop taking it. There are other prescription medications that will increase the flow of urine without reducing prostate size. They tend to work within a couple of days. You could use a medication to increase flow while you are waiting for the other medication to shrink the gland. You should discuss your options with your doctor.

3   Saw palmetto may reduce the amount of PSA in the blood and interfere with the PSA test used to detect prostate cancer. Please tell your doctor if you are taking saw palmetto.

4   Many people can reduce the chance of urinary tract infections by drinking lots of fluid and increasing the amount of urine they make. Men with enlarged prostate glands who get infections will not benefit from this.

5   Sitting down to urinate may make the whole experience easier for you. This gives you more time to urinate and allows you to relax more. Take your time and be patient -- you may empty more urine if you wait after the initial pause of urine flow. Sitting down to pee will also make your spouse happier that the lid is down and you haven't created the usual splash zone!

Problems with Urination: WOMEN

SUMMARY: Unlike men, women do not have a prostate gland. They also have a much shorter distance between the bladder and the skin. This shorter tube is called the urethra. In youth, the urethra is on an angle to reduce the chances of the bladder emptying on its own. With age and the experience of childbirth, there is a tendency for this angle to straighten. So, while men tend to experience problems with decreased urine flow, women tend to have problems with urinary incontinence. Urinary incontinence is simply the passage of urine when you are not planning on doing it. About 15% of seniors will have a bladder control problem. Don't worry—treatment exists.

Possible Symptoms:

▸ need to rush to the bathroom
▸ loss of small amounts of urine with coughing, laughing or sneezing
▸ increased number or urination episodes per day
▸ burning discomfort with urination
▸ large volume urine loss

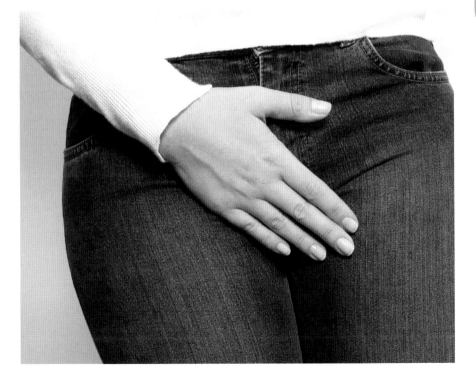

Problems with Urination

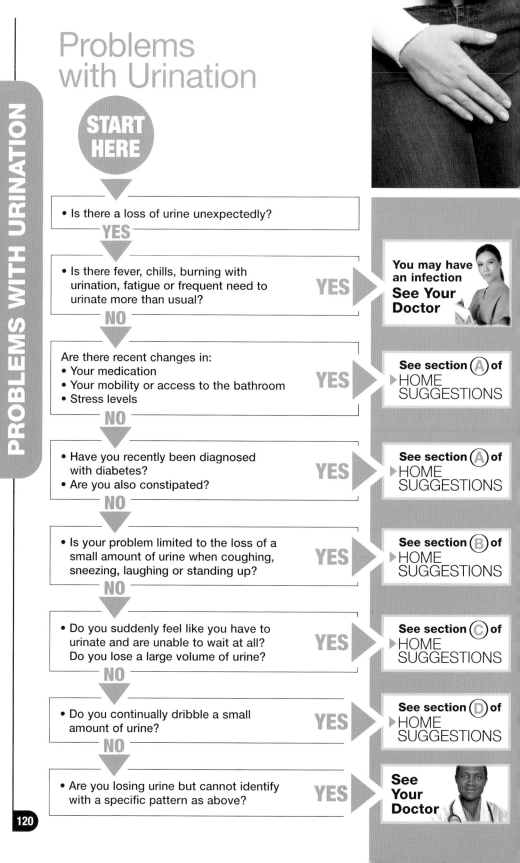

START HERE

- Is there a loss of urine unexpectedly?

YES

- Is there fever, chills, burning with urination, fatigue or frequent need to urinate more than usual?

YES → You may have an infection **See Your Doctor**

NO

Are there recent changes in:
- Your medication
- Your mobility or access to the bathroom
- Stress levels

YES → See section (A) of ▶HOME SUGGESTIONS

NO

- Have you recently been diagnosed with diabetes?
- Are you also constipated?

YES → See section (A) of ▶HOME SUGGESTIONS

NO

- Is your problem limited to the loss of a small amount of urine when coughing, sneezing, laughing or standing up?

YES → See section (B) of ▶HOME SUGGESTIONS

NO

- Do you suddenly feel like you have to urinate and are unable to wait at all? Do you lose a large volume of urine?

YES → See section (C) of ▶HOME SUGGESTIONS

NO

- Do you continually dribble a small amount of urine?

YES → See section (D) of ▶HOME SUGGESTIONS

NO

- Are you losing urine but cannot identify with a specific pattern as above?

YES → **See Your Doctor**

▶ HOME SUGGESTIONS

(A) Medications

There are many medications that can affect your ability to control your urination. These can be either non-prescription or prescription medications. Some of the most common medications that may cause problems include: sleeping pills, anti-inflammatory painkillers, tranquilizers, high blood pressure pills, cough and cold medications and diuretics (pills designed to make you urinate more for the purpose of treating conditions such as high blood pressure or congestive heart failure). Occasionally medications used to treat depression, other mental illnesses or Parkinson's disease may disturb bladder function. If your doctor has prescribed a new medicine or changed the dose, you may wish to talk to them about this new problem. If the recent change is with a new non-prescription medicine, you could talk to your pharmacist about an alternative.

Mobility

Consider if you have had a recent change or restriction of your ability to get up and around due to a location change, an illness or injury. This will often result in a transient loss of the ability to control urination. Often, with time, the situation normalizes and the incontinence goes away.

Constipation

Constipation or stool impaction can be a problem in the elderly, especially if you are drinking less than usual. Constipation can affect your bladder function and cause incontinence. Remember that decreasing your fluid intake so that you will not have to urinate will only make this worse. When the constipation is relieved, the bladder will often function normally again. It is advisable that you eat a high fiber diet.

Depression or Anxiety

If you have recently been depressed or have been overstressed, you may temporarily have a problem with bladder control. Moving to a new home, losing a loved one or being separated from lifelong friends or family may cause many to suffer disruption in their usually stable functions. Your doctor may be able to help you with these problems. When symptoms of depression or anxiety improve, we often see an improvement in bladder function.

Diabetes or Hormonal Dysfunction

Diabetes causes increases in blood sugar and urine volumes. Some illnesses may cause increases in calcium levels. Occasionally the first sign of these disorders may be a change in urinary control. Your doctor can help determine if you have developed one of these diseases. If you are diabetic getting good control over your blood sugar can reduce the incontinence problem.

continued next page...

▶ HOME SUGGESTIONS

(B) This is usually called Stress Incontinence and results from increased pressure in the abdomen that causes a small amount of urine to be squeezed out of your bladder. This can occur because the muscles under your bladder are weak. Medications can also cause a similar problem. If you have had a recent medication change (especially in blood pressure medications), this should be discussed with your doctor. This problem can also be aggravated or caused by a chronic cough. There are exercises that can successfully strengthen the pelvic muscles that are necessary to squeeze the bladder valve shut (see the section on Kegel exercises, next page). Estrogen can also be of help to women by re-vitalizing the tissues in the genital area. If these exercises don't help, we suggest you talk to your doctor about medicines that help tighten the valve at the base of your bladder. A surgical treatment, called bladder suspension, is sometimes needed to control these symptoms.

(C) This is usually called Urge Incontinence and results from a sudden spasm of the bladder. The most simple home treatment is to empty your bladder frequently, whether you feel the need to or not. It is best if you put yourself on a schedule. You can also try bladder training: when you feel the urge to urinate, go directly to the bathroom but once you are there, try and hold it until the urge passes. The more you can train the bladder to tolerate the spasms, the fewer problems you will have. If the condition persists, you need to discuss this with your doctor to find the cause and try other treatments.

(D) This is called Overflow Incontinence and results when the outflow of the bladder is obstructed and the muscle of your bladder is not working well. Your bladder is always full and is constantly leaking out the excess volume which it cannot possibly hold. It is like running water into a pail that is already full -- the added water simply overflows. Diabetes and some medications may cause this type of incontinence. You should urinate on a regular basis, whether it feels like you need to or not. If an obstruction is the problem, removal of the obstruction is necessary. A change in medication may also help. If the muscle of your bladder no longer functions to squeeze the urine out, you may need to keep the bladder completely empty for a few days by having a catheter inserted. Please discuss this problem with your doctor.

▶ GENERAL SUGGESTIONS

1   Stay active. Don't let this upset your enjoyment of life and the things you love to do. Use the available products such as **Depends** to help you continue to do everything that is important to you. If you let this ruin your life, your incontinence will likely just get worse due to increased stress.

2   Try and develop a regular habit of urinating at a frequency that minimizes your incontinence.

3   Try "double voiding." This is when you empty your bladder, relax for a minute or two, and then try again. This can result in more complete emptying of your bladder. Have a book or a magazine handy.

4   Avoid drinks that have caffeine in them (coffee, tea, cola soft drinks, etc.). It is also advisable to avoid liquids for three to four hours before going to bed to help minimize the need to have to get up in the night. Do not decrease your overall liquid intake.

5   When you are away from home, make sure that you dress in clothes that make it easy to urinate in a hurry.

Kegel exercises for stress incontinence

These exercises are easily performed and can be done almost anywhere once you get the hang of them. They work to build up the muscles that are important in controlling the flow of urine.

You can easily get the feel of which muscles you must squeeze by practising this exercise when you are urinating. The next time you are urinating, squeeze in a way that makes you suddenly stop, then release and let the urine flow again. Repeat. You do not need to tighten your stomach, buttocks or your leg muscles, just those in your pelvis around your urethra and your anus. It can be reassuring to do this with each time you urinate to show yourself that you can actually stop your urine if you want to.

Once you have learned how to do this easily, you can do it almost anywhere, sitting or standing. Squeeze the muscles for a count of five and then release and relax for a count of five. Do this in a set of 15 to 20 squeezes. Repeat the whole set of exercises three or four times a day. You can greatly benefit from this few minutes of exercise each day. Some experts suggest mixing in sets of long sustained squeezes of 10 seconds or even sets of rapid alternating contractions and relaxations. Squeeze, relax, squeeze, relax, squeeze, relax and so on. None of these exercises are better than others. It is most important that you try some or all of them to see how you do. Remember that this is a long-term project and must be continued for life.

Sexual Dysfunction: MEN

SUMMARY: To have successful sexual relations, you first must have desire and then you must have the equipment. For many men the desire is present, but they are let down by erectile dysfunction. A successful erection is one that is of sufficient firmness to allow penetration and lasts long enough to complete the sexual act. A dysfunction of the erectile function of the penis is not a sign of weakness, nor a loss of manliness. For many, this problem is related to a deterioration of the nerves and blood vessels that serve the penis. For some, it is a side-effect of medication. For many, there may be treatment available.

Men who can develop an erection with some women but not others do not have erectile dysfunction. Some men are under stress, are depressed, or are nervous about sexual activity. This can result in an inability to achieve an erection. Feeling wanted and sexually attractive are also factors. If you are worried that you are unattractive to your partner, you may not be able to have an erection.

Possible Symptoms:

▸ Inability to develop an erection
▸ Inability to maintain an erection

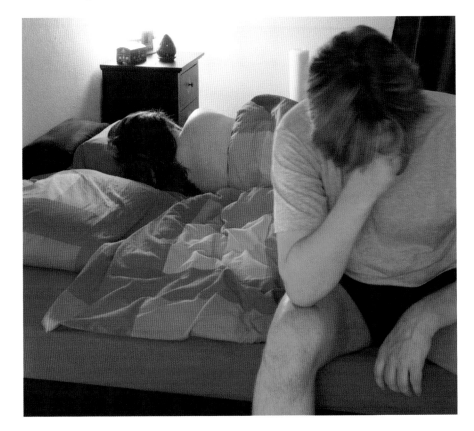

Sexual Dysfunction

MEN

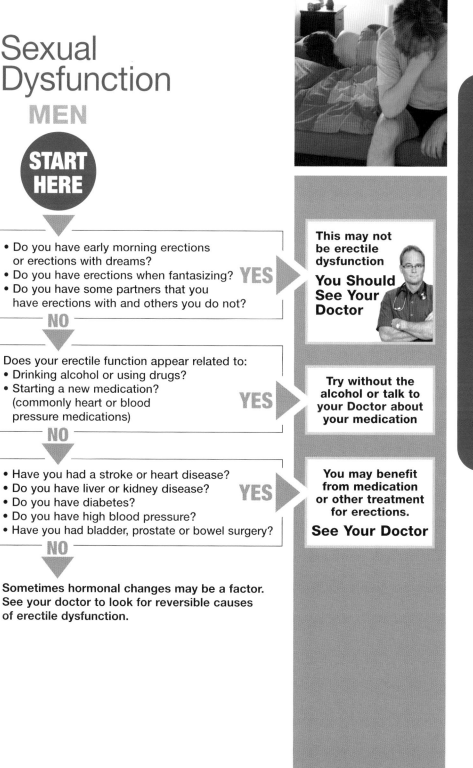

START HERE

- Do you have early morning erections or erections with dreams?
- Do you have erections when fantasizing?
- Do you have some partners that you have erections with and others you do not?

YES → This may not be erectile dysfunction

You Should See Your Doctor

NO

Does your erectile function appear related to:
- Drinking alcohol or using drugs?
- Starting a new medication? (commonly heart or blood pressure medications)

YES → **Try without the alcohol or talk to your Doctor about your medication**

NO

- Have you had a stroke or heart disease?
- Do you have liver or kidney disease?
- Do you have diabetes?
- Do you have high blood pressure?
- Have you had bladder, prostate or bowel surgery?

YES → **You may benefit from medication or other treatment for erections.**

See Your Doctor

NO

Sometimes hormonal changes may be a factor. See your doctor to look for reversible causes of erectile dysfunction.

Sexual Dysfunction: WOMEN

Sexual dysfunction in women is complicated.
There are four areas of dysfunction.

DESIRE: There may be a loss of desire in comparison to previous level

AROUSAL: When you don't feel your body responding or maintaining a sexual arousal

ORGASM: When you can't attain orgasm

PAIN: When sexual activity results in pain.

All women recognize the difference between their needs for sexual activity and those of their partners. Comfort in the relationship, stresses in the house, fatigue, looking after a home and children may all reduce desire. Intimacy prior to bed and a connection with your spouse are powerful players in desire and arousal. Coming to bed after the game for sex might be okay for guys but often is a non-starter for women.

Depending on the cause of the dysfunction there may be specific treatment to help.

Occasional problems with sex are not evidence of a disease. Many women may find sex sometimes does not feel good. This does not mean you have a problem. However, if you never want sex or if it never feels good, you might have a problem. Talk to your doctor. Remember they are trained for this purpose.

1   To improve desire, you might try different times of the day or positions.

2   If you have vaginal dryness you can try lubricants or estrogen creams.

3   Reaching orgasm may be enhanced with masturbation, extra stimulation with a vibrator or your partner may have to gently stroke your clitoris. Sometimes it can take several minutes to an hour to reach orgasm. This does not mean you have a problem.

4   If sexual activity is painful, make sure you empty your bladder before intercourse. Try different positions. Slower initial penetration may be better tolerated. Woman on top might be easier. Using lubricants or having a bath before intercourse may make penetration less painful.

5   For some woman, the addition of estrogen, or the male hormone testosterone may improve libido (sexual desire). Even **Viagra** has been used to improve female desire. See your doctor to discuss the pros and cons.

Topics for All Ages

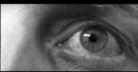
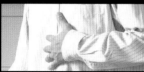
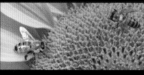
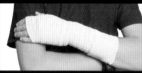
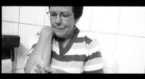
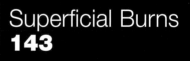
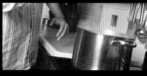
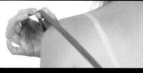
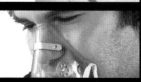

Conjunctivitis
or "Pink Eye"

SUMMARY: "Pink eye" is an irritation of the white of the eye and the eyelid. It can make your eye look red or pinkish in colour. It is easily passed from person to person. Thorough handwashing by both the sufferer and the caretaker is very important to prevent the spread of infection.

Often when someone is suffering from pink eye their eyes will make more tears. This can make the eyes uncomfortable and crusty after sleep. Clean the crusts away by holding a warm, damp cloth gently over the eye. Recheck the eye about an hour later. If there is just a small quantity of crusty discharge, then the cause of this eye irritation is likely viral. If, however, a creamy, runny or stringy discharge is forming then the cause is probably bacterial. Conjunctivitis is irritating but should not be too painful. If there is a lot of pain, you should see your doctor. Follow the instructions in **HOME SUGGESTIONS** and you should be able to take care of this illness at home.

Please note: During the allergy season (spring through fall), a very itchy eye most likely indicates an allergic reaction rather than pink eye.

ALL AGES
Possible Symptoms:

Affecting one or both eyes

▸ red eyes
▸ swollen lids
▸ itchiness

▸ crusting or pussy eyes
▸ gritty eyes
▸ increased tearing

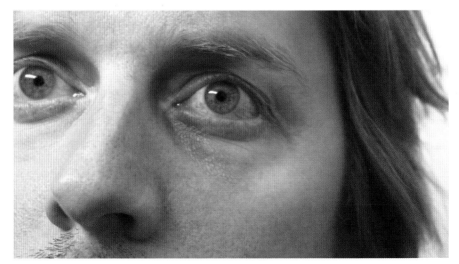

Conjunctivitis
or "Pink Eye"
ALL AGES

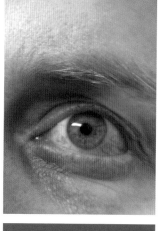

START HERE

PINK EYE

- Is there severe redness or swelling around the eye?
  or
- Is there pain around or behind the eye or is there pain with eye movements?
  or
- Is there a fever present? (see page 94)
  or
- Are you having trouble seeing?
  or
- Is this a newborn child?
  or
- Has there been recent eye surgery?
  or
- Do you wear contact lenses?
  or
- Does bright light hurt the eyes?
  or
- Have you noticed the pupils are different sizes?

YES ▶

Use acetaminophen, ibuprofen, or ASA for pain (see page 58) and then,

GO TO THE HEALTH CENTRE *or* **HOSPITAL NOW** **H**

NO

60 minutes after cleaning your eyes with warm water and a cloth, is there (choose one)...

A creamy discharge from the eye?

A crusty discharge from the eye?

See **HOME SUGGESTIONS A** (see page 130)

See **HOME SUGGESTIONS B** (see page 130)

Start again from the top of this chart every 6 to 8 hours

If not better within 48 to 72 hours **YES** ▶

GO TO THE HEALTH CENTRE *or* **HOSPITAL**

Conjunctivitis or "Pink Eye"
ALL AGES

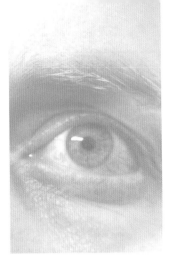

▶ # HOME SUGGESTIONS

Suggestions (A)

1   Try a non-prescription antibiotic drop such as **Polysporin**. Place 2 drops in the "pink" eye four times daily. Continue this treatment for 7 days. If the eye is not improving after 3 days you should see your doctor.

2   Clean the eye with a warm cloth as necessary.

3   Warm or cool cloths put on the eye for 20 minutes at a time may soothe the discomfort, pressure and swelling. Use whatever seems to work the best for you.

4   Avoid smoke and other things which bother your eyes.

5   Avoid wearing contact lenses until your eye has been normal for 2 to 3 days.

Suggestions (B)

1   Non-prescription decongestant eye drops, such as **Visine** or **Vasocon**, can help soothe the eye. Those with severe heart disease or poorly controlled blood pressure should avoid decongestant medications. See page 176 for more details about decongestant medications. Ask your pharmacist for help in choosing these medications.

2   Clean the eye with a warm cloth as necessary.

3   Avoid smoke and other things which bother your eyes.

4   If there is severe itching, there may be an allergy causing the problem. Antihistamine pills or antihistamine containing eye drops may help. See page 177 for more details about antihistamines. Ask your pharmacist for help in selecting these medicines.

5   Avoid wearing contact lenses until your eye has been normal for 2 to 3 days.

Heartburn

SUMMARY: Heartburn is a burning discomfort felt behind the breastbone. This discomfort is made worse by meals, bending over or lying down. Fatty foods, spicy foods, peppermint, coffee, alcohol and cigarette smoking may also cause heartburn. Almost 90% of the population will get heartburn from time to time. Many people, however, will have episodes of heartburn more often. Those who suffer from severe or frequent heartburn may need regular medication to control symptoms. Anyone who has heartburn and difficulty swallowing should see their doctor. Sometimes heartburn can be increased by prescription medicines. If you have started a new medicine and have been suffering with heartburn, please see your doctor. Use the flowchart to help you decide if you should see your doctor.

ALL AGES
Possible Symptoms:

▶ burning discomfort behind the breastbone (increased by bending over, lying down and eating)

▶ regurgitation of food and a sour taste in the mouth (especially on bending over)

▶ associated symptoms may include bloating after meals

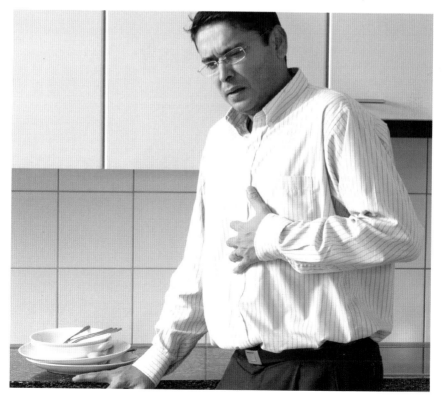

Heartburn
ALL AGES

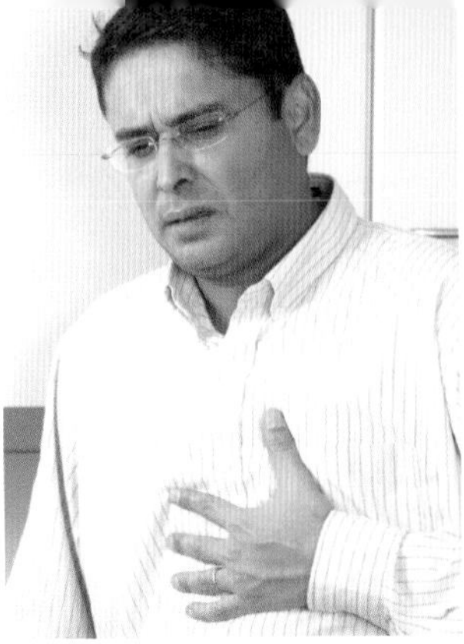

START HERE

HEARTBURN

- Is there any sweating, vomiting, shortness of breath, dizziness or chest tightness?
  or
- Have you passed bloody or thick black bowel movements?
  or
- Have you vomited blood?

YES → **GO TO THE HEALTH CENTRE or HOSPITAL NOW** [H]

NO

Try an antacid
See **HOME SUGGESTIONS**

- Has the severe or new heartburn continued for over 10 minutes after a dose of antacid? **YES** → **GO TO THE HEALTH CENTRE or HOSPITAL NOW** [H]

NO

- Have you had unexpected weight loss?
  or
- Does food stick on the way down after swallowing?
  or
- Do you have heartburn more than 3 times per week?

YES → **GO TO THE HEALTH CENTRE or HOSPITAL**

NO

See **HOME SUGGESTIONS**

- Do you still have symptoms after 2 to 4 weeks of treatment? **YES** → **GO TO THE HEALTH CENTRE or HOSPITAL**

NO

Continue therapy.

▶HOME SUGGESTIONS

1   Antacids are non-prescription (over-the-counter) products, which neutralize acid. They are available in liquid and tablet form. They may contain magnesium hydroxide (which may cause diarrhea), aluminum hydroxide (which may cause constipation) or calcium carbonate (**Tums**, **Rolaids** and others). Antacids may contain a mixture of magnesium and aluminum (**Maalox** or **Riopan** for example) to reduce any side-effects. You can take antacids when you want rapid relief of heartburn. There will not be any long-lasting effect. If taken regularly after meals or at bedtime then they may help prevent or reduce your heartburn discomfort. If you need to take antacids more than twice a day then you should see your doctor.

2   Medicines containing alginic acid, such as **Gaviscon**, may prevent heartburn symptoms when taken after meals or at bedtime. This medicine is not a true antacid, but creates a barrier which prevents the acid coming back up from your stomach.

3   You can help yourself feel better by making some changes to your daily habits:
   • do not lie down for 2 hours after meals
   • do not eat within 2 hours of bedtime
   • raise or elevate the head of your bed 6 inches on blocks. Propping yourself with pillows won't be as helpful and may actually cause more trouble.
   • cut back or eliminate your caffeine intake. Caffeine is found in coffee, tea, chocolate and most cola drinks
   • cut back or eliminate your use of alcohol and cigarettes
   • cut back your use of ASA and anti-inflammatory medication if possible. Try acetaminophen (**Tylenol** and others) instead
   • cut back your intake of fatty foods: high fat meats, fried foods, gravy and sauces
   • spicy foods and peppermint often cause heartburn
   • if a food causes you discomfort, avoid eating it a second time.

4   Some medications may increase heartburn symptoms. If you develop new symptoms after starting a new medication consult your doctor.

5   Also available without a prescription are the acid-reducing drugs cimetidine (**Tagamet**), ranitidine (**Zantac**), famotidine (**Pepcid**) and nizatidine (**Axid**). These medications are also available in higher strengths as prescription medications. If you try one of these medications and find that it does not give you complete relief of symptoms or that you require regular or prolonged use of these drugs to feel well, you should discuss this with your doctor.

HEARTBURN

Bee Stings or Insect Bites

SUMMARY: Most insect bites and stings cause reactions at the site of the bite or sting. The discomfort of these bites is usually easy to relieve and treat at home. The use of cold compresses and antihistamines will help significantly.

ALL AGES
Possible Symptoms:

minor and localized

▸ pain
▸ redness
▸ swelling

major or severe (anaphylaxis)

▸ shortness of breath
▸ swelling of the mouth, tongue, or throat
▸ light-headedness or dizziness
▸ severe rash over large areas

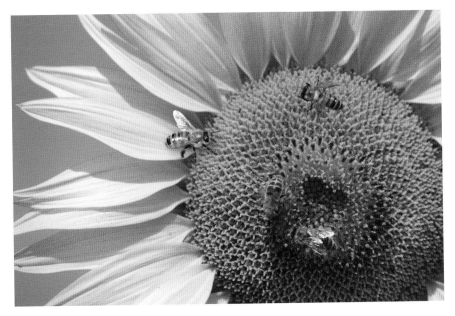

Bee Stings or Insect Bites
ALL AGES

START
HERE

BEE STINGS OR INSECT BITES
You have been bitten or stung by an insect (bee, wasp, hornet, mosquito, blackfly, etc.).

- Do you have difficulty breathing?
  or
- Do you have mouth or throat swelling?
  or
- Are you severely light-headed or dizzy?
  or
- Do you have a history of a previous severe reaction to insect bites or stings?

YES ▶ If available: Use adrenalin kit and take antihistamine pill. Then, **GO TO THE HEALTH CENTRE** or **HOSPITAL NOW** [H]

NO

- Are there a large number of stings? (greater than 10 stings from bees, hornets, wasps etc.)

YES ▶ **GO TO THE HEALTH CENTRE** or **HOSPITAL NOW** [H]

NO

See **HOME SUGGESTIONS**

AFTER 48 HOURS:
- Is there a fever, increasing redness or red streaking up a limb?

YES ▶ **GO TO THE HEALTH CENTRE** or **HOSPITAL**

NO

See **HOME SUGGESTIONS**

If any symptoms develop after 7 to 10 days

YES ▶ **GO TO THE HEALTH CENTRE** or **HOSPITAL**

135

Bee Stings or Insect Bites
ALL AGES

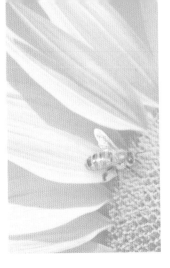

▶ HOME SUGGESTIONS

1   If you have previously had an allergic reaction to a sting or bite you should immediately take an antihistamine (see page 177). If you do not have a known allergy you should wait for redness, swelling or itching to develop and take an antihistamine to relieve these symptoms if they occur.

2   Apply a cold pack immediately for a maximum of 20 minutes, which will reduce the redness and swelling. You can reapply this cold pack for 20 minutes every hour as long as there is redness and swelling.

3   In relieving the discomfort of a sting it is important to make sure you have removed the stinger. At the end of the stinger there is a venom sack which can continue to release venom as long as it is embedded in the skin. To remove the stinger you should gently scrape it out from the side with a sharp-edged object like a knife. Do not squeeze and pull.

4   Non-prescription or over-the-counter antihistamine or hydrocortisone cream can help reduce the skin irritation and itch. Ask your pharmacist to help you choose this medicine.

5   If you have had a serious reaction in the past you should carry an adrenaline kit with you. Discuss this with your doctor.

Strains and Sprains of the Limbs

SUMMARY: Strained muscles and sprained ligaments are commonly the result of over-use, sports activity or trauma—playing a sport on an occasional basis is the most common cause. Using R.I.C.E.: Rest, Ice, Compression, Elevation immediately will help speed your recovery. These "soft tissue" injuries should slowly improve over a period of 1 week. Returning to regular activity too early may prolong an injury. Be aware that early in the day may be one of the most difficult times due to the stiffness that can develop as a result of being inactive throughout the night. Give yourself time to improve over the morning hours.

ALL AGES
Possible Symptoms:

▶ pain and tenderness in the joint or muscle

▶ swelling and redness of a joint or muscle

▶ bruising around a joint or muscle

▶ difficulty moving a joint or muscle

Strains and Sprains of the Limbs
ALL AGES

START HERE

POSSIBLE LIGAMENT SPRAIN OR MUSCLE STRAIN

- You cannot stand on your injured leg?
  or
- You cannot bend your joint normally?
  or
- Is there obvious deformity of the joint or limb?
  or
- Is the skin cut or scraped over the area?

YES → Use pain medication (acetaminophen, ASA, ibuprofen, etc.) and **GO TO THE HEALTH CENTRE** or **HOSPITAL NOW** **H**

NO

See **HOME SUGGESTIONS**

- Is the pain still bad after using HOME SUGGESTIONS?

YES → **GO TO THE HEALTH CENTRE** or **HOSPITAL**

NO

Over the first 48 hours
- Is there increasing swelling or redness despite treatment?
  or
- Is it remaining difficult to move the joint?
  or
- Is there continued severe pain?

YES → **GO TO THE HEALTH CENTRE** or **HOSPITAL**

NO

Continue **HOME SUGGESTIONS**

- Is the muscle or joint function still abnormal or is there significant pain after 1 week?

YES → **GO TO THE HEALTH CENTRE** or **HOSPITAL**

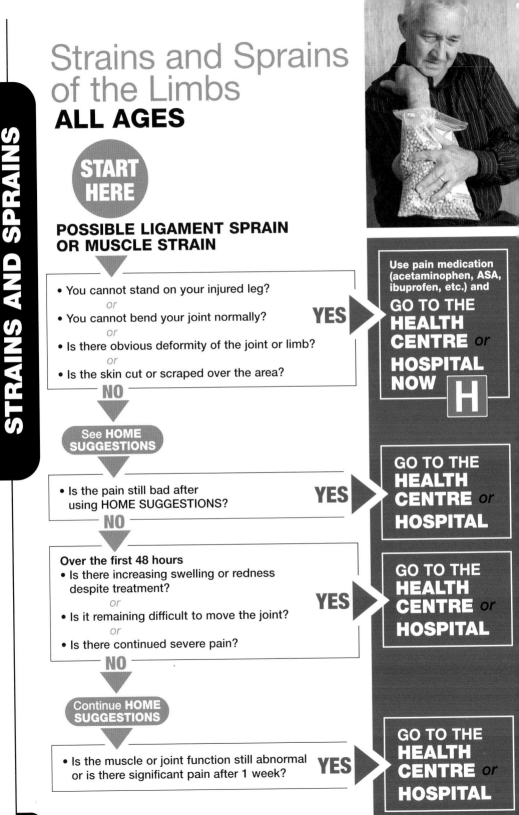

ALL AGES

▶HOME SUGGESTIONS

1   R.I.C.E. REST, ICE, COMPRESSION, ELEVATION
Rest the area for the first 48 hours. After this time your body will let you know how much you should be doing. Using a sling or crutches may be helpful.

Ice is used to reduce swelling. Apply ice, cold packs, or even frozen peas or corn for proper shaping to your injured area. Start by applying the ice for 20 minutes on, 20 minutes off, for the first 2 hours. Thereafter use ice 5 times daily for the first 2 days. To prevent frostbite, protect your bare skin from icy materials by wrapping them in a towel.

Use an elastic bandage to wrap areas of swelling. You can also use these type of bandages for support.

Elevation of a limb will help reduce swelling. Place your arm in a sling or elevate your foot or leg on a pillow.

2   After the first 48 hours you can continue with ice or switch to heat therapy. Use whatever makes you feel better. You may find that alternating between cold and hot therapy feels good. You should not use heat during the first 48 hours because it may increase swelling. Remember to protect bare skin from hot water bottles etc. to prevent burns by putting the hot water bottles into a towel.

3   After 48 hours begin to move the injured area but avoid anything causing serious pain.

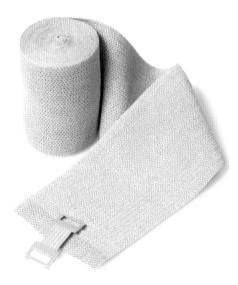

Scrapes and Abrasions

SUMMARY: Scrapes and abrasions are very common and easily treated at home. If the area affected is large, deeply injured or appears infected, you should see a doctor. Treatment depends on good initial cleaning and watching for infection. Most scrapes or abrasion will heal in 1 to 2 weeks.

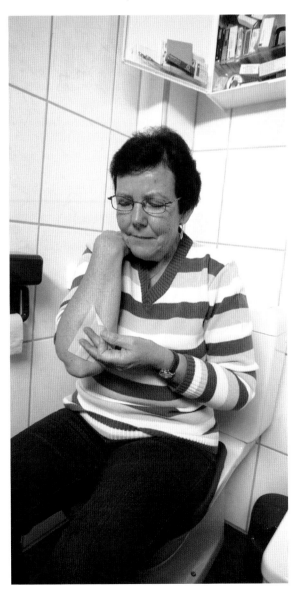

ALL AGES

Possible Symptoms:

▶ scraped skin that may or may not bleed

▶ dirt in the abrasion

▶ not a cut, the skin is not spread apart

Scrapes and Abrasions
ALL AGES

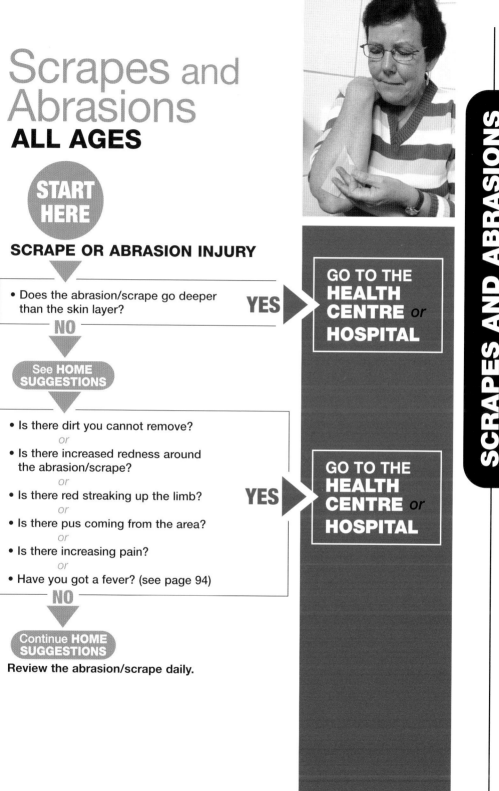

START HERE

SCRAPE OR ABRASION INJURY

▼

- Does the abrasion/scrape go deeper than the skin layer? — **YES** ▶ GO TO THE **HEALTH CENTRE** or **HOSPITAL**

— **NO** —

▼

See **HOME SUGGESTIONS**

▼

- Is there dirt you cannot remove?
  or
- Is there increased redness around the abrasion/scrape?
  or
- Is there red streaking up the limb?
  or
- Is there pus coming from the area?
  or
- Is there increasing pain?
  or
- Have you got a fever? (see page 94)

YES ▶ GO TO THE **HEALTH CENTRE** or **HOSPITAL**

— **NO** —

▼

Continue **HOME SUGGESTIONS**

Review the abrasion/scrape daily.

Scrapes and Abrasions
ALL AGES

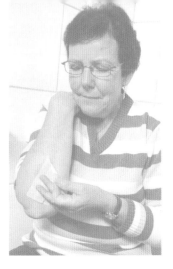

▶ HOME
SUGGESTIONS

1   Wash the abrasion with warm water. Letting water run over the area is best. If discomfort prevents you from doing this then soak the scraped area with warm wet cloths. You may need to scrub the area to remove dirt. You may repeat the washing as many times as necessary to clean the scraped area thoroughly. Clean water and soap is all you really need to do this.

2   If pain prevents cleaning all the material out of the abrasion you should use a local anaesthetic like **Bactine** to make the process less painful.

3   Take acetaminophin (**Tylenol** and others), ASA (**Aspirin** and others) or ibuprofen (**Advil**, **Motrin**, and others) for pain. Do not give ASA to anyone under 20 years of age. See page 178 for details.

4   We suggest you apply an antibiotic ointment (**Polysporin** and others) 2 or 3 times daily and cover the abrasion with a bandage, gauze or non-stick **Telfa**. Use enough ointment to prevent the bandage from sticking to the injured skin. Covering the abrasion may speed healing and keep the area clean.

5   You should check that you have had a tetanus boost immunization in the last 10 years. If not you should see your doctor. The last regularly scheduled immunization is usually at age 14.

Superficial Burns

SUMMARY: Small burns even if blistered can be treated at home. Burns must be cleaned and kept clean. Using simple soap and warm water is all that is needed. It is important to reassess your burn as it can change over time. Minor burns should heal within 1 to 2 weeks.

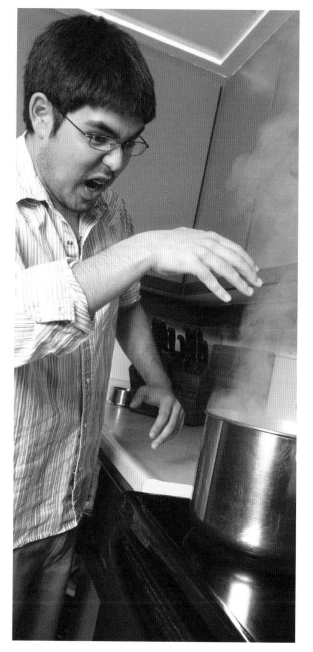

ALL AGES

Possible
Symptoms:

▶ redness
▶ tenderness
▶ pain
▶ swelling
▶ blistering

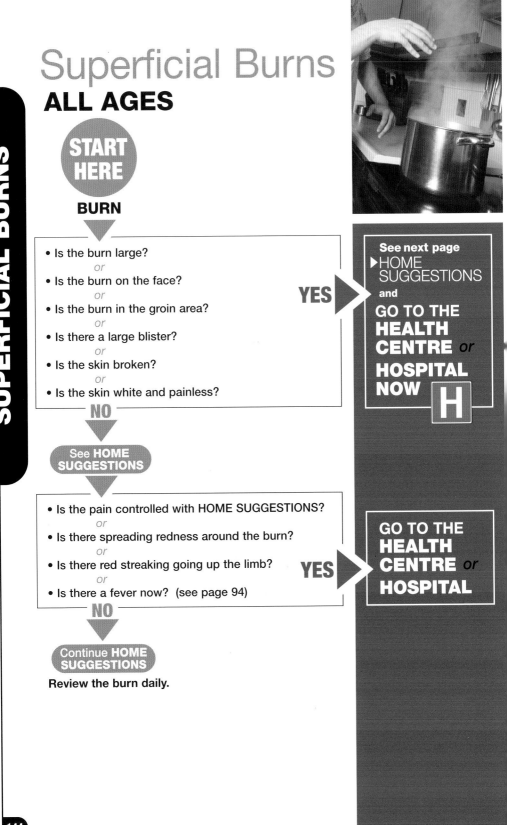

Superficial Burns
ALL AGES

START HERE

BURN

- Is the burn large?
  or
- Is the burn on the face?
  or
- Is the burn in the groin area?
  or
- Is there a large blister?
  or
- Is the skin broken?
  or
- Is the skin white and painless?

NO

See **HOME SUGGESTIONS**

- Is the pain controlled with HOME SUGGESTIONS?
  or
- Is there spreading redness around the burn?
  or
- Is there red streaking going up the limb?
  or
- Is there a fever now? (see page 94)

NO

Continue **HOME SUGGESTIONS**

Review the burn daily.

YES →
See next page
▶ HOME SUGGESTIONS
and
GO TO THE HEALTH CENTRE *or* **HOSPITAL NOW** **H**

YES →
GO TO THE HEALTH CENTRE *or* **HOSPITAL**

Superficial Burns
ALL AGES

▶HOME SUGGESTIONS

1   Immediately place the burned area into cold water or apply a cold compress for 10 to 15 minutes. This will cool the hot skin and reduce further injury.

2   Burned skin must be kept clean. Wash it with soap and water. Putting some local anaesthetic like **Bactine** or benzocaine (**Solarcaine**) on the burn may allow you to clean and dress the burn with less pain.

3   If a blister breaks apply an antibiotic ointment (**Polysporin** and others) and cover with a bandage, gauze or non-stick **Telfa**. Apply enough ointment to prevent the bandage from sticking to the injured skin.

4   If the skin is unbroken you can apply a moisturizing skin cream 3 times daily. Some of these may contain aloe, a natural healing substance.

5   If a burned area is throbbing you may feel better if you elevate it. Place your arm in a sling or your foot on a pillow.

6   If you do not have stomach problems you could use an anti-inflammatory pain medication like ASA (**Aspirin** and others) or ibuprofen (**Advil**, **Motrin**, and others). See page 58 for more details. Do not use ASA (**Aspirin** and others) in anyone under 20 years of age.

SUPERFICIAL BURNS

Sunburn

SUMMARY: Sunburns are similar to other burns caused by hot objects. Sunburns cover larger areas of skin but are usually minor burns. They are commonly associated with chills, fever and may be associated with dehydration. Treatment of a burn includes cooling the skin, controlling the discomfort and protecting the skin from further injury. Watch for dehydration (sunstroke). Burning and tanning both increase your risk of skin cancer. There is no such thing as a good burn. Please remember to use sunscreen. Be sure to put sunscreen on children even if they are going out for only short periods of time. It usually takes only 20 to 30 minutes to burn in the summer.

ALL AGES
Possible Symptoms:

▶ red tender skin

▶ blistered skin

▶ fever or chills

▶ dehydration
   (see Ⓐ page 77 for children or page 112 for adults)

▶ flaking, itching, tingling skin

▶ sunstroke (page 148)

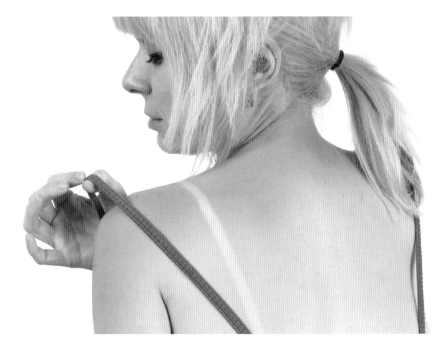

Sunburn
ALL AGES

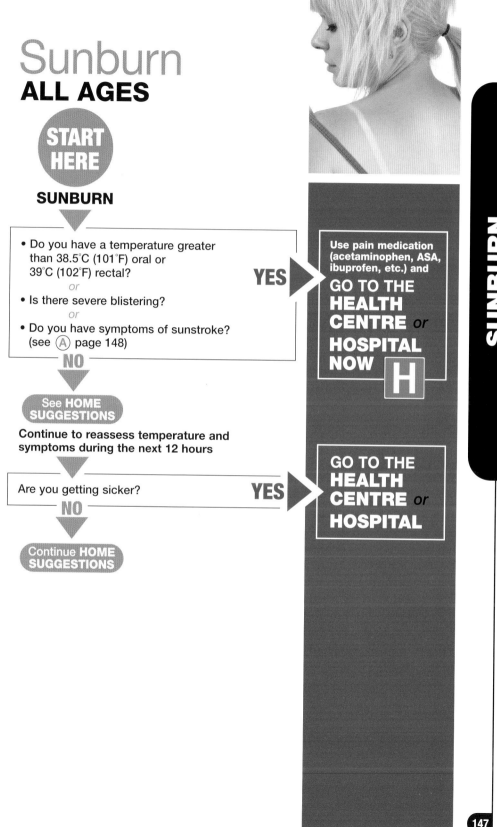

START HERE

SUNBURN

▼

- Do you have a temperature greater than 38.5°C (101°F) oral or 39°C (102°F) rectal?
  or
- Is there severe blistering?
  or
- Do you have symptoms of sunstroke? (see Ⓐ page 148)

NO
▼

See **HOME SUGGESTIONS**

Continue to reassess temperature and symptoms during the next 12 hours

▼

Are you getting sicker?

NO
▼

Continue **HOME SUGGESTIONS**

YES ▶

Use pain medication (acetaminophen, ASA, ibuprofen, etc.) and

GO TO THE HEALTH CENTRE *or* **HOSPITAL NOW** Ⓗ

YES ▶

GO TO THE HEALTH CENTRE *or* **HOSPITAL**

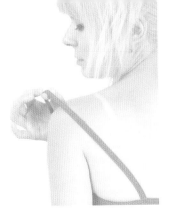

Sunburn
ALL AGES

▶ # HOME SUGGESTIONS

Ⓐ Symptoms of dehydration and sunstroke

- temperature greater 39°C (102°F) rectal or 38.5°C (101°F) oral
- heart rate greater than 100 beats per minute at rest
- no sweating
- light-headed when you stand
- confusion
- muscle cramps
- passing out
- headache
- nausea and vomiting

All of the above symptoms may develop more quickly when the victim has also been drinking alcohol.

Therapy for sunburn

1 Cool the burned skin with a cold bath, damp towel or cold shower.

2 Drink plenty of non-alcoholic fluids.

3 Apply a moisturizing cream to the burned area liberally, several times daily.

4 Use acetaminophen (**Tylenol** and others), ASA (**Aspirin** and others) or ibuprofen (**Advil**, **Motrin** and others) for pain and fever control. Do not give ASA to those under 20 years of age. See page 178 for details.

5 Painful skin may be treated with local anaesthetic spray or ointments such as benzocaine (**Solarcaine**).

6 Stinging or itching can be treated with 0.5% hydrocortisone which is available without a prescription.

7 Antihistamines may reduce itching. See page 177 for details.

8 Don't expose burned skin to the sun even with sunscreen applied. Wear a hat, long sleeves and long pants.

9 Always wear a hat and apply a sunblock 30 or higher to prevent sunburn. Apply sunblock liberally to children.

SUNBURN

Shortness of Breath

One of the most distressing sensations you can suffer is shortness of breath—the sense that you just can't get enough air can be almost painful. Lung function is vital and fortunately we are born with more lung function than we really need. Loss of lung function can occur as a result of age, lung damage or injury. Sometimes the loss of function is temporary and reversible, as in conditions such as asthma or as a result of infection; sometimes the changes are permanent, such as those seen in smokers.

With every breath you take, you breathe in oxygen and breathe out carbon dioxide. The oxygen is used to power the cells of your body and the carbon dioxide is produced as exhaust. Shortness of breath is due to either a reduction of oxygen levels in your body, or an increase in carbon dioxide levels that are normally responsible for you wanting to breathe. Anything that interferes with the movement of air in and out of your lungs reduces your ability to move oxygen into your blood and carbon dioxide out of your blood, and you will become short of breath.

This section will deal with the most common causes of shortness of breath. Sometimes people may have more than one reason at the same time.

ASTHMA

Asthma is the most common chronic condition seen in children and accounts for a lot of the shortness of breath seen in adolescents and adults. It may also complicate other conditions, such as smoking-induced lung damage (COPD), heart disease and pneumonia.

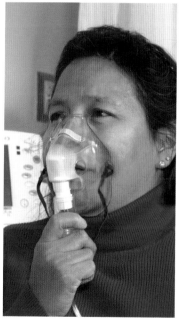

To illustrate how asthma affects breathing, think of this simple example. It is easier to blow through a pipe than a straw; the narrower the opening, the more difficult it is to blow air. In asthma, the airways become narrower due to swelling and spasm of the muscle that controls their size. The result is noisy or wheezy breathing and more difficulty moving air in and out of the lungs. Although asthma may make breathing very difficult, the changes are temporary and can completely resolve with treatment.

Asthma attacks may be triggered by many things. Allergies, infection, exercise, cold air, stress, and smoke are common triggers. Some people get attacks of asthma for no obvious reason.

The treatment of asthma includes avoiding known triggers and using medication that reduces swelling or relaxes muscle to open spastic airways. Often people have to go the emergency department for treatment but many can treat attacks at home with the right medications.

See the following section specifically for Asthmatics.

continued next page...

Shortness of Breath

Smokers Lung Chronic Obstructive Pulmonary Disease (COPD)

Many people are afraid of smoking because it increases their risk of lung cancer. Although this is true, the real danger of smoking is the slow but progressive damage to the microscopic areas of the lung where oxygen and carbon dioxide are exchanged. Many smokers start at a young age when they have much more lung function than they will ever use. As time progresses, however, there is a slow but permanent loss of function because of smoke damage.

Eventually the smoker begins to notice a change in his ability to breathe. They may get short of breath more quickly with activity that would have previously caused no symptoms. By this time, the changes are very severe and may not be reversible. Although people who have COPD can use medications to improve function, ongoing exposure to cigarette smoke will eventually cause too much damage. Many people in this situation may need supplemental oxygen to be able to get around. Higher carbon dioxide levels affect how your brain and heart work.

Congestive Heart Failure

When people have suffered damage to the heart muscle or the heart valves, the heart may not be able to move blood as easily. This can result in back pressure. Fluid can accumulate in the lungs, collecting in the tissue separating the air channels of the lung from the blood channels and making the movement of oxygen and carbon dioxide into and out of the blood more difficult. Eventually the oxygen levels in the blood fall, affecting all parts of your body.

Treatment of congestive heart failure includes medications to reduce the amount of fluid, to improve the pumping of the heart and to reduce the chance of further heart damage. Sometimes damaged heart valves have to be repaired or replaced.

Pneumonia

Pneumonia means an infection of the lung. Lung infections can be of viral or bacterial origin. While we do not have medications that can treat most viral infections, bacteria may respond to antibiotics. There is also a vaccination for the most common cause of adult bacterial pneumonia. Ask your doctor.

When the lung is infected, it becomes swollen and may stop working. If you have limited lung function due to previous damage or if a large amount of lung is involved in the infection, you may be short of breath. Pneumonia is often accompanied by fever and sweats, cough with or without sputum, and pain on breathing. Please see your doctor or go to hospital if you believe you have pneumonia.

Shortness of Breath
ALL AGES

START HERE

SHORTNESS OF BREATH

- Are you a known asthmatic? **YES** ▶ See section **A** of HOME SUGGESTIONS

NO

- Are you a long-time smoker? **YES** ▶ See section **B** of HOME SUGGESTIONS

NO

- Do you have known heart failure? **YES** ▶ See section **C** of HOME SUGGESTIONS

NO

- Do you have associated chest pain or pressure?
- Does it hurt to breath?
- Do you have a temperature over 38.5°C (101°F) oral / 39°C (102°F) rectal?
- Have you recently developed swelling of your feet or legs?
- Are you light-headed or have you fainted?
- Is there bluish discolouration of fingers, toes or lips?

YES ▶ **GO TO THE HOSPITAL NOW H**

NO

- Are you making a wheezing sound? **YES** ▶ You may have asthma, see Asthma Section. **GO TO THE HEALTH CENTRE or HOSPITAL**

NO

- Are these symptoms new today? **YES** ▶ **GO TO THE HOSPITAL NOW H**

NO

- Are these mild or slowly changing symptoms? **YES** ▶ **GO TO THE HEALTH CENTRE or HOSPITAL**

Shortness of Breath

ALL AGES

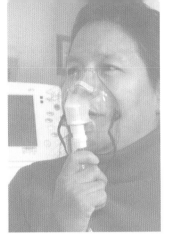

▶ ## HOME SUGGESTIONS

HOME SUGGESTIONS (A)

1   Remove yourself or your family member from the trigger area or avoid the trigger substance as soon as possible. The trigger may be a substance to which you are allergic (pollen, pet, dust mites in a bed, smoke, polluted air, perfume, aspirin), it may be air temperature (very hot or cold), it may be because of exercise, it may be a stress.

2   If you have **Ventolin** (salbutamol) or **Bricanyl** (terbutaline), use it immediately. If you do not get relief or improvement within 10 minutes, take another dose and go to hospital.

3   If you are on inhaled corticosteroids, make sure you are taking your medication correctly.

4   If attacks are occurring more frequently, than see your doctor about adjustment of your medication to reduce attacks.

5   See the following section on Asthma.

HOME SUGGESTIONS (B)

Smokers are at risk of developing minor infections which may reduce lung function for a short period of time. Signs of these infections include an increase or change in the colour, quantity or taste of the phlegm coughed up and increasing wheezing. These infections may not be severe enough to cause fever. Exacerbations of COPD may respond to an increase in regular medications such as **Ventolin** and **Atrovent** and the addition of antibiotics and anti-inflammatory steroids. You may take an additional dose of your bronchodilator mediations and YOU SHOULD SEE YOUR DOCTOR.

HOME SUGGESTIONS (C)

If you have a history of congestive heart failure you may also have a history of heart attack and angina. Increasing difficulty with heart failure may mean that you are having more angina. If you wear a nitro patch and it is not on, put it on now. If you are having chest pain you should take nitroglycerin under your tongue. You should chew two 81mg **Aspirin** tablets. If you normally take diuretics or water pills, take an additional dose now. If you do not improve or if you are deteriorating within 20 to 30 minutes, go to hospital.

Asthma

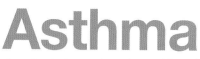

Imagine being underwater and breathing through a garden hose, then being given a small straw to breathe through. You would have to work much harder to get the air in and out through the smaller tube.

This is similar to what happens in your lungs during an asthma attack. Your airways are tubes that run into your lungs and swelling on the inside of the tubes can narrow the opening. In addition, muscle in the walls of the airways can spasm and squeeze them tighter. This is what makes an asthmatic huff and puff while they are having an attack. If not treated, the inflammation can cause permanent damage to the lungs, as well as increase the risk of future asthmatic attacks.

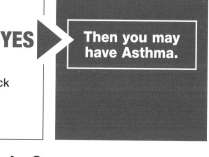

DO YOU EXPERIENCE...

▼

- Feeling breathless
- Working hard to breathe
- A tight chest
- Wheezing (high pitched or whistling sound when you breathe)
- A dry cough that is not related to being sick
- Frequent night cough
- Shortness of breath after 5 to 20 minutes of exercise

YES ▶ **Then you may have Asthma.**

What causes asthma attacks?

The following is a list of items that can cause asthma attacks. This means that it is also a list of items that many asthmatics should avoid, although every asthmatic person may not have a problem with every item.

- The common cold
- Tobacco smoke
- Pet dander
- Dust and dust mites
- Mold
- Pollen and seasonal allergies
- Cold air
- Perfume
- Certain foods
- Air pollution
- **Aspirin**

▶HOME SUGGESTIONS

- Make sure you follow the personal Asthma Action Plan that you should receive from your doctor and use your medicines exactly as prescribed.
- Learn to use a "peak flow meter" to monitor your asthma.
- Never smoke and avoid smoky areas.
- Cover pillows and mattresses in airtight covers to reduce exposure to dust mites.
- Avoid all the items (listed above) that you know can possibly cause an asthma attack.
- Avoid having pets in the home or at least in the bedroom.
- Remove carpets and drapes, especially from the bedroom.
- Spray the carpets that remain to get rid of dust mites.
- Keep the humidity below 50% in your home.

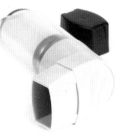

Asthma
ALL AGES

You Must Understand Your Asthma Medicine

There are two categories of medicine used in the control of asthma: short-term rescue medications and long-term controllers. They are usually taken via a "puffer". Puffers may be difficult for some people to work properly; ensure that you receive training in the correct technique from a knowledgeable healthcare professional.

Rescue Medicines

Rescue medicines provide immediate relief from the symptoms of an asthma attack. They are designed to relax spasms in the muscles in your airways. They work immediately at the time of the attack, but do not treat the underlying cause, so do not prevent future attacks. In Canada, the most common rescue medicines are salbutamol (**Ventolin**) and terbutaline (**Bricanyl**).

Controller Medicines

These medicines work to decrease inflammation on a continuous basis and therefore prevent future attacks. The most important of these medicines are **Inhaled Corticosteroids** (ICS). As the name suggests, these medicines contain steroids, which are anti-inflammatory medications that work to reduce the swelling of the airways in order to prevent symptoms and prevent long-term damage to your lungs.

A basic rule of thumb for evaluating the use of your asthmatic medications is: If you need to use a rescue puffer more than three times a week or have symptoms of night cough, you need to increase the dose of your controller medicine. A personalized "Asthma Action Plan" should give precise guidelines on how to do this and when.

Exercise Induced Asthma (EIA)

Many asthmatics suffer attacks shortly after they start to exercise, especially if they are breathing in air pollution or cold air. For some, this is the only time that they have asthma symptoms. These asthmatics have symptoms as a result of spastic airway muscle contraction alone and do not have inflammation. These individuals can avoid attacks by using a rescue medication, such as salbutamol, 15 to 20 minutes before exercise. Other asthmatics will need to either take a rescue medication before exercise, or increase the dosage of their controller medication (corticosteroid) to prevent airway spasm by controlling inflammation that complicates muscle spasm during exercise. It is also advised that you warm up slowly as you start to exercise.

 It is important to remember that poorly treated, long-term asthma can cause permanent damage.

Emotional or Mental Health

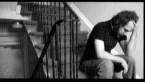
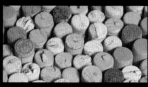
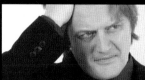
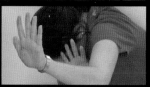
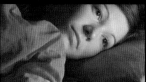
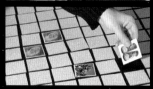
EMOTIONAL OR MENTAL HEALTH

Emotional or Mental Health Issues

Introduction

There are several common psychiatric and emotional problems that affect people's day-to-day lives, and about one in five patients attending doctors' offices will have a mental health problem. Frequently, these problems are not dealt with because people have other symptoms that they want dealt with first. Commonly, these patients don't realize how these mental health issues may affect how they cope with other diseases and how they may be related to their symptoms.

Having a mental health disorder is not a sign of weakness. Many psychiatric disorders develop as a result of an imbalance of the chemicals that make the nerve cells in our brains work properly. Just as the person who does not make or use insulin properly will develop diabetes, the person who does not make or use the chemicals that control their mood properly may develop depression. Commonly these disorders start with mild symptoms and minor disorders of the nerves. If we address these problems early, they are easier to reverse.

This section of our book is designed to help you or your loved ones:

- decide if symptoms observed might be related to a mental disorder
- manage these symptoms at home during the early stages
- decide if you should be seeing your doctor about these symptoms
- understand more about mental health disorders

Most of the symptoms of mental health disorders involve normal feelings or emotions. A mental disorder is present when these feelings or emotions become too strong, too frequent or interfere with our ability to lead a normal life. They may interfere with our ability to work, play or continue our relationships with family or friends. The vast majority of these disorders involve mood (depression), worry (anxiety) or substance abuse (alcohol, drugs).

We recommend that you read all of these sections, but you can turn to the one that is most likely to be associated with your present concern at any time.

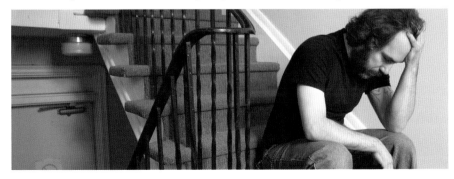

Disorders of Mood
Depression

Possible Symptoms:

- ▶ prolonged low mood or sadness
- ▶ lack of pleasure or interest in life
- ▶ decreased energy or intense fatigue
- ▶ loss of appetite and weight loss
- ▶ early awakening from sleep, can't get to sleep
- ▶ loss of sex drive
- ▶ loss of confidence, poor self-image
- ▶ intense feelings of guilt
- ▶ inability to concentrate
- ▶ thoughts of suicide

SUMMARY: Depression is the medical term used to describe one of the disorders of mood. Depression usually means too much sadness or an intense sensation of feeling down. There are those among us who have the opposite mental disorder. Mania refers to the condition in which someone may feel so good that they do not realize the consequences of their behaviour. They may spend all their money and get deeply into debt. They may have energy to work all night. Most patients with mania will swing over to severe depression (bipolar disorder).

Everyone has experienced sadness or lack of energy from time to time. Often these feelings are the result of a big change in our lives, such as a loss like the death of a loved one, a failed relationship or the loss of job. One can also suffer depression after giving birth or as a result of substance abuse. Most of the time we get over these feelings and carry on. If these feelings are so intense that they interfere with normal living or working, or if they last too long or occur for most of the day, this may suggest that the person is suffering from a mental disorder.

Depression is the most common mental disorder, affecting 1 in 50 people at some time in their lives. The good news is that early recognition, counselling and often prescription medication can cure and prevent further episodes of depression.

If depression is very severe, it may result in a person feeling that there is no way they can go on living. They may attempt to commit suicide or develop problems with substance abuse. We know that if we can identify those who are depressed early, we may prevent some of these complications.

The following chart can help you decide if you or your loved one are suffering from depression.

Disorders of Mood
Depression

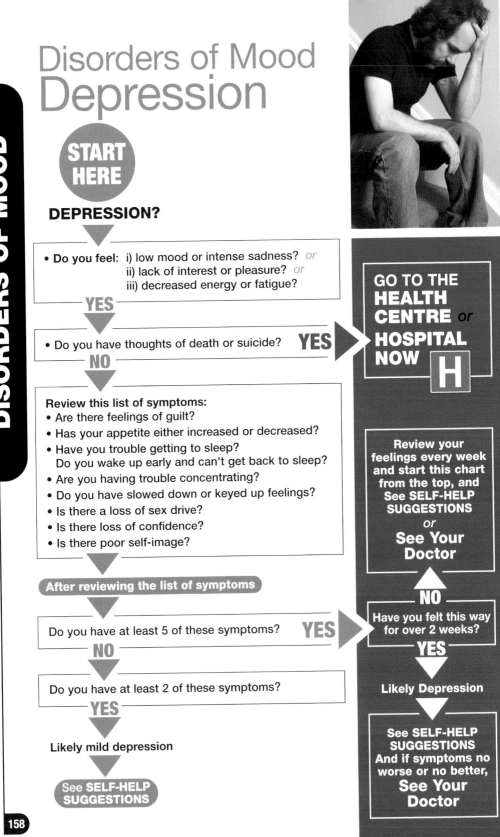

START HERE

DEPRESSION?

- **Do you feel:** i) low mood or intense sadness? *or*
  ii) lack of interest or pleasure? *or*
  iii) decreased energy or fatigue?

YES

- Do you have thoughts of death or suicide? **YES** → **GO TO THE HEALTH CENTRE** *or* **HOSPITAL NOW** **H**

NO

Review this list of symptoms:
- Are there feelings of guilt?
- Has your appetite either increased or decreased?
- Have you trouble getting to sleep?
  Do you wake up early and can't get back to sleep?
- Are you having trouble concentrating?
- Do you have slowed down or keyed up feelings?
- Is there a loss of sex drive?
- Is there loss of confidence?
- Is there poor self-image?

After reviewing the list of symptoms

Do you have at least 5 of these symptoms? **YES** →

NO

Do you have at least 2 of these symptoms?

YES

Likely mild depression

See SELF-HELP SUGGESTIONS

Review your feelings every week and start this chart from the top, and **See SELF-HELP SUGGESTIONS** *or* **See Your Doctor**

NO

Have you felt this way for over 2 weeks?

YES

Likely Depression

See SELF-HELP SUGGESTIONS And if symptoms no worse or no better, **See Your Doctor**

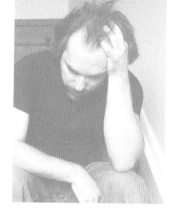

▶SELF-HELP SUGGESTIONS

1. Make a list of your feelings and how bad they are. Rate them as mild, moderate or severe. See the list on the previous pages to help.
2. Look for the trigger or change that may have started your depression (job change, move, etc.). Can it be "fixed"? Discuss this with a close friend, family member, counsellor, nurse or doctor.
3. Think about options to deal with the trigger (for example get a new job).
4. Try to take small steps towards a solution. (Are there other jobs available?)
5. Write down things that you usually enjoy and do more of them.
6. Stop negative thoughts when they appear, and try to think more positively.
7. Eat a proper diet.
8. Go to bed on time and try to get your sleep.
9. Make yourself do physical exercise. Start with a 15 to 20-minute brisk walk every day.
10. Seek out other resources to help you cope. See your doctor for counselling or a referral.

Other treatment information

Although depression is often triggered by a change or loss, it is still an illness caused by an imbalance in the chemicals or hormones in the brain that regulate mood. Sometimes we need to use medication to correct this imbalance. This is similar to treating diabetes by giving patients insulin or giving patients with reduced thyroid function thyroid hormone replacement.

If you are prescribed antidepressant medications, you should take them every day as prescribed. You should not change the dosage or stop the medication unless you discuss this with your doctor or nurse. Unfortunately, these medications do not work overnight and may take as long as 6 weeks to start helping.

Side-effects of modern antidepressants are rare, but sometimes a specific medication may not be the right one for you. If you suffer side-effects, be sure to tell your doctor. Sometimes we have to try alternatives to find one that works well without side-effects. It is most likely that you will have to take them for several months before you and your doctor decide to change. Antidepressants are not "uppers" and are not addictive. They will have little effect on those without the chemical imbalance of depression.

Counselling is another helpful tool in the treatment of depression. It can be used with or without medication. Counsellors are trained to help you make your depression better by helping you understand how you can affect your mood and improve those situations that cause you to feel depressed.

Remember that alcohol and other drugs may make it harder to treat depression and can counteract the benefits of antidepressant medications. Please let your doctor know if you are using alcohol or other drugs.

Substance Abuse and Addictive Behaviours

SUMMARY: The medical and social effects of substance abuse do not have anything to do with whether a substance is legal (alcohol, cigarettes) or illegal (cocaine). Abuse refers to the use of a product in a manner that negatively affects the performance of the normal activities of daily living. Addiction usually implies that someone cannot live without using the substance, that is they will suffer some physical or mental discomfort on withdrawal.

Some abuses and addictions are worse than others. Alcohol is by far the most abused substance that we have in North America. Cigarette smoke is probably the worse substance for addiction. Generally we do not think that people who smoke tobacco are abusing tobacco. Unfortunately, some abuse of alcohol and drugs is seen as a lifestyle choice. Addiction is usually seen as a true medical illness.

Since alcohol is a substance that is commonly abused and is associated with addiction, we will use alcohol as our example in the following pages. There are many other substances that people can consider when answering our questions. Many people who either abuse or become addicted to one substance or another do so because they believe the use of these substances will help them to deal with other medical or mental disorders. People who abuse drugs or alcohol are not bad or weak. We should always try to look for the underlying reason for substance abuse.

Possible Symptoms:

▶ unable to use alcohol without becoming intoxicated
▶ have lost a job, driver's licence or have been hospitalized because of drug or alcohol use
▶ cannot resist the urge to drink or take drugs
▶ suffer physical symptoms if you do not take drugs or drink alcohol
▶ have been told that you are abusing alcohol or drugs

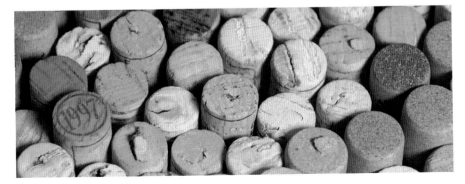

Substance Abuse and Addictive Behaviours

ADDICTIVE BEHAVIOUR

You may be addicted if you note any of the following when you do not take alcohol or drugs.

Psychological Symptoms

sleeping problems
trouble concentrating
increased anxiety
decreased appetite

Physical Symptoms

poor energy/fatigue
stomach pains, nausea,
weight loss

You may be suffering alcohol/drug dependence if you have the following:

Psychological

sleeping problems
trouble concentrating
low mood
increased anxiety/stress

Physical

falls
blackouts
poor energy or fatigue
increased blood pressure
increased weight
stomach complaints

You may be addicted or dependent on alcohol/drugs if you experience:

Problems with relationships, have frequent fights or arguments

Problems with fulfilling work, school, or home responsibilities

Problems with the police or you have been arrested because of alcohol or drug use

Withdrawal from relationships or responsibilities

ALCOHOL ABUSE

Are you at risk?

Men

Do you drink more than 3 drinks per day or 21 drinks per week?

Women

Do you drink more than 2 drinks per day or 14 drinks per week?

A drink is 1 beer, or 1oz of liquor, or 4oz of wine

Have you?

- not been able to stop, decrease or control drinking
- not been able to resist the urge to drink
- had physical problems when you stop drinking i.e. sweats, shakes, fast heartbeat, headaches, poor sleep, seizures, restlessness
- kept drinking even though you knew it was causing a problem
- been told by anyone you have a drinking problem

If you answered yes to any of the above you have a drinking problem.

Substance Abuse and Addictive Behaviours

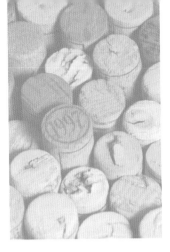

SELF-HELP SUGGESTIONS

1   Set a goal for reduced intake. The acceptable intake for men is no more than 3 drinks per day and women 2 drinks per day. Give yourself 2 non-drinking days per week.

Do not drink if you are:
   pregnant
   developing a physical problem
   driving, exercising or working

Act to reach your goals.
   • keep track of how much you are drinking
   • dilute your drinks
   • drink non-alcoholic drinks before every alcoholic drink
   • delay time of day for first drink
   • decide on 2 non-drinking days
   • avoid places with alcohol
   • eat when drinking alcohol

2   Get help. Search out support groups such as AA. Discuss the problem with family and friends. See your doctor for assistance.

If you know someone who has a problem with an addictive substance, you can make the most impact by confronting them with the problem and suggesting that they seek help. Trying to help them cover up the problem may only contribute to the addictive behaviour. Addictive behaviour can lead to physical and verbal abuse problems that put you in danger. If you live with someone who has a problem with substance abuse, you may also need help. Talk to your doctor or counsellor. Often friends and family are helpful for support, but may not know how to deal with the situation any better than you.

Abuse or addiction may occur with over-the-counter medications, prescription drugs or illegal drugs. It may occur with many other substances such as glue, paint or gasoline, which can be sniffed. Addictive behavior may also involve activities such as gambling. As a general rule of thumb, if a behavior is repetitive and interferes with one's ability to carry on the normal activities of daily living, it is a potential addiction. See your doctor to discuss this problem further. Our self-help suggestions for alcohol may be modified for other substances or behaviours.

If you need more information about how to help yourself or a loved one who may have an addiction problem please contact your doctor, local health unit or the community mental health unit in your area.

Anxiety Disorders

SUMMARY: It is normal to feel the worry or tension of a fearful or threatening situation. What can be abnormal is to experience excessive worry, tension or fear in situations where there would normally be no reason for these feelings. When these feelings interfere with normal daily activities or relationships, then one is said to have an anxiety disorder. People who suffer from anxiety disorders should receive some treatment.

Many of these people realize that something is wrong with their feelings. They may describe themselves as going crazy or losing their minds. This is not a weakness of character or a personality problem. These anxiety disorders are common, may present in varying degrees of severity and can be treated if identified. Review the flow chart to see if you or a loved one may be suffering from an anxiety disorder.

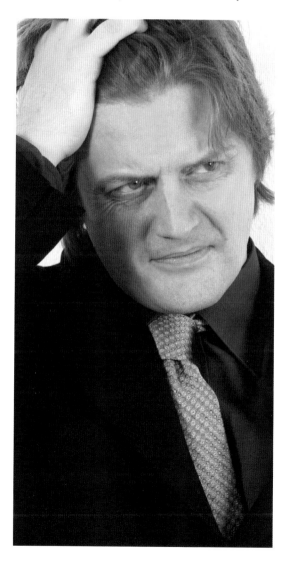

Possible Symptoms:

Psychological
▶ worry
▶ fear of losing control
▶ fear of going crazy
▶ fear of dying

Physical
▶ trembling
▶ sweating inappropriately
▶ heart pounding
▶ dizziness
▶ shortness of breath
▶ light-headedness
▶ muscle soreness
▶ numbness/tingling
▶ stomach problems

Anxiety Disorders

START HERE

ANXIETY DISORDER

▼

Do you • feel tense or upset?
        • worry a lot?

YES ▼

Do you experience?
- worry
- fear of losing control
- fear of going crazy
- fear of dying
- trembling
- sweating
- heart pounding
- dizziness
- light-headedness
- muscle soreness
- shortness of breath
- stomach pains, nausea, vomiting
- numbness, tingling

YES ▼

- Do your symptoms interfere with school, work, relationships or other normal activities?
- Do your symptoms occur out of proportion to the situation?
- Do your symptoms occur often?

YES ▼

See **SELF-HELP SUGGESTIONS** ▶

- Do you experience sudden fear "out of the blue" for no reason?

NO

YES

Continue to use SELF-HELP SUGGESTIONS, and See Your Doctor

▲

You may have a General Anxiety Disorder

You may have a Panic Disorder

▼

Continue to use SELF HELP SUGGESTIONS, and See Your Doctor

Anxiety disorders affect some people all the time and others only under specific circumstances. Extreme symptoms can result in a panic attack. We all experience panic at some time, which is a natural defense against danger. When this happens for no apparent reason, however, it is a very unpleasant feeling. Chemicals in our brains control the panic response. If these chemicals are released at the wrong time a panic attack may occur. Anxiety and panic attacks can be treated—they are not a sign of weakness.

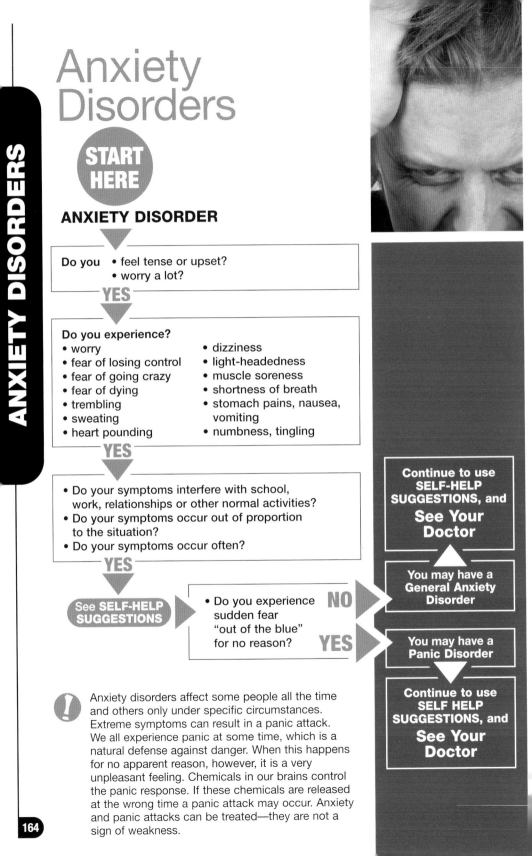

Anxiety Disorders

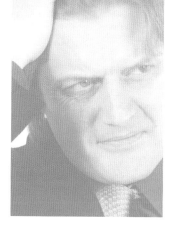

▶ # SELF-HELP SUGGESTIONS

- Recognize symptoms of anxiety/panic may be treated.
- Look for triggers such as:
  - too much alcohol, caffeine
  - lack of sleep
  - relationship problems, including abuse
  - taking on too much
  - physical illness
  - a recent loss
- Set goals to manage triggers.
- Identify your fears (ie. public speaking).
- Take small steps to confront your fears
  (i.e. try to speak in front of 1 or 2 friends you feel comfortable with).
- Seek help from friends, family, primary care provider, support groups.
- Try to treat symptoms: Physical symptoms of light-headedness, tingling,
  numbness, and shortness of breath are commonly due to hyperventilation.
  You can concentrate on slow deep breaths or breathe into a paper bag.
  See Breathing exercises below.

Medication and other treatment

For severe symptoms, medication is often prescribed. Some of these medications can be addictive and often lose their effectiveness with prolonged use. Many of these medications have similar chemistry to diazepam (**Valium**). Side-effects are common and need to be discussed with your doctor.

Counselling and behaviour modification therapy are the best long-term approaches to anxiety disorders. Talk to your primary care provider about this approach.

Breathing exercises

- Breathe in for 3 seconds then out for 3 seconds then pause for 3 seconds
  before you take another breath in
- Practice this for 10 minutes morning and night
- Use before and during situations that cause anxious feelings for you
- During the day, make a point of checking and slowing down your breathing

Psychotic Illness

SUMMARY: Unlike the mental health disorders discussed above, which involve problems with feelings and emotions, psychotic illnesses are disorders of thought. Schizophrenia is the most common psychotic disorder. It is not multiple personalities.

Psychotic disorders usually occur for no specific reason, but they can run in families and may be a result of drug abuse or even a side-effect of some prescription medications. People with psychotic disorders often do not think they have a problem. They often become paranoid and think that the rest of the world is the problem or that everyone else is against them. As a result, they will not seek help voluntarily. If you think someone has a psychotic disorder they should be evaluated by a trained mental health provider or a doctor. If the person will not do so voluntarily, it may be necessary to have them seen against their will. This is best arranged through the police, a justice of the peace or a physician. Psychotic disorders are very serious and there is a really no place for self-help other than to get the person to a clinic or hospital where they can be evaluated. Fortunately, as with most mental health disorders, the root of the problem is a chemical imbalance in the brain. As a result, these disorders can be treated by medications that correct this imbalance.

Possible Symptoms:

▶ withdrawal/isolation from friends and family
▶ hallucinations—hearing voices, seeing things
▶ speech problems
▶ less attention to hygiene/dress
▶ inability to do school work or perform at work
▶ strange thoughts especially of outside control
▶ unusual behaviours especially directed from outside

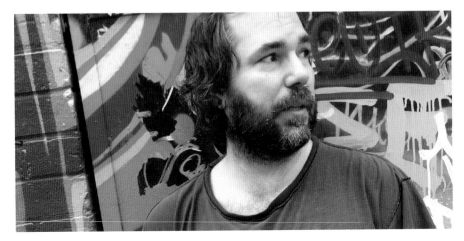

Domestic Violence and Abuse

SUMMARY: The most difficult aspect of human relationships to understand is how and why we take advantage of those closest to us. When this reaches an extreme it is abuse. Abuse can happen between partners or be directed at childen. It may be verbal, physical or sexual. Often the victims of abuse blame themselves, which prevents them from escaping the situation and may in fact increase the abuse. Abuse is never acceptable. The only answer is to leave the situation and make yourself safe.

It is possible for a person not to understand that their actions toward another are abusive. We hope this section will help both the abuser and the victim of abuse realize what may be happening.

Have you experienced?

▶ name-calling, insults and putdowns
▶ isolation from friends or family
▶ physical attacks, such as slapping, punching, biting, kicking
▶ threats with a weapon
▶ forced sex
▶ being prevented from getting a job or doing activities outside the home
▶ threats of harm to you, your children or pets

If you have, then you are victim of abuse and need to get away and get help!

Have you been guilty of or caused?

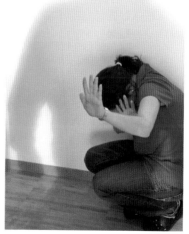

▶ name-calling, insults, and putdowns
▶ isolation from friends or family
▶ physical attacks, such as slapping, punching, biting, kicking
▶ threats with a weapon
▶ forced sex
▶ someone to not get a job or do activities outside the house
▶ threats of harm to you, your children, or pets

If you have, then you are an abuser and need to get help.

Domestic Violence and Abuse

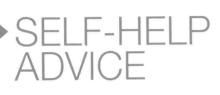

▶ SELF-HELP ADVICE

Victim

Safety comes first

1 Leave - options include
   - hospital emergency
   - safe homes, shelter (Interval house)
   - Salvation Army

2 You have choices
   - the police do not need to be involved
   - counselling may help

Abuser

Admitting there is a problem is the first step

1 Remove yourself form the environment

2 Change is necessary, counselling may help. Consult:
   - your doctor
   - community health centre
   - private counselling

No form of abuse is acceptable under any circumstances. Abuse will end only if a zero tolerance position is adopted. Assault programs can help with safety planning, risk assessment and referrals to a "safe house". Help with transportation to medical care and counselling can be provided. Assistance to access legal services is also provided.

Problems with Sleep

SUMMARY: There are many different sleep problems and problems with sleep can be part of many different medical and mental health conditions. The most common sleep problem is insomnia. This may be described as a problem getting to sleep, or a problem with staying asleep.

How much sleep a person needs is variable. Most adults sleep about 7 to 8 hours each night. Many people seem well with much less sleep. Some need more to feel well. The total number of hours of sleep one gets is less important than how one feels after sleeping. A lack of daytime tiredness and a sense of refreshment after sleep are signs of adequate sleep.

Sleep patterns may change with age. Those over 60 often note they sleep less and that their sleep is more interrupted. This is normal. A similar pattern may be seen in babies. Treatment is not necessary as long as the person feels well. Reasurrance is all that is necessary in most cases.

A sleep problem may lead to mental or physical problems as outlined in the possible symptoms above.

Use the following chart to help you determine if you have a sleep problem and whether you should be seeking professional advice.

Possible Symptoms:

▶ difficulty getting to sleep even though you are tired

▶ difficulty staying asleep

▶ falling asleep during the day

▶ trouble concentrating

▶ trouble with memory

▶ inability to make decisions or do your job

▶ increased injuries or accidents (i.e. car accidents)

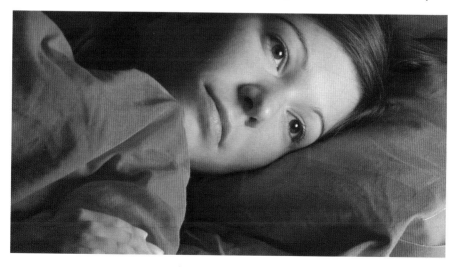

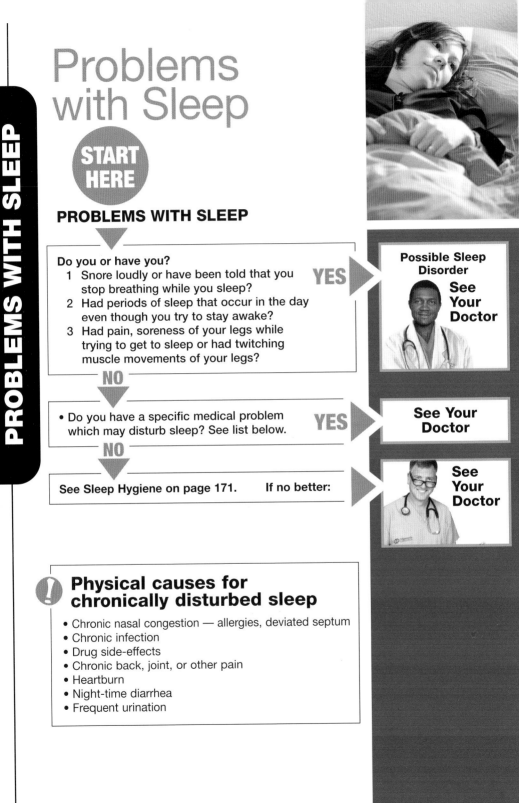

Problems with Sleep

START HERE

PROBLEMS WITH SLEEP

▼

Do you or have you?
1. Snore loudly or have been told that you stop breathing while you sleep?
2. Had periods of sleep that occur in the day even though you try to stay awake?
3. Had pain, soreness of your legs while trying to get to sleep or had twitching muscle movements of your legs?

YES ▶ **Possible Sleep Disorder**
See Your Doctor

NO ▼

• Do you have a specific medical problem which may disturb sleep? See list below. **YES** ▶ **See Your Doctor**

NO ▼

See Sleep Hygiene on page 171.　　If no better: ▶ **See Your Doctor**

❗ Physical causes for chronically disturbed sleep

- Chronic nasal congestion — allergies, deviated septum
- Chronic infection
- Drug side-effects
- Chronic back, joint, or other pain
- Heartburn
- Night-time diarrhea
- Frequent urination

Problems
with Sleep

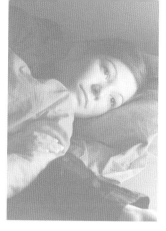

▶ SELF-HELP SUGGESTIONS

1 Try to determine the cause of your sleep problem
CONSIDER
- A specific sleep disorder (See flowchart page 170)
- Physical problem (See list page 170)
- Emotional problem - depression, anxiety, stress (See specific sections page 158)
- Environmental problems - too noisy, too light
- Lifestyle problems - excessive alcohol, coffee, nicotine, shift work, daytime naps, inadequate exercise, or too much late evening exercise

2 Sleep hygiene
- Improve sleep habits by trying to go to bed and arising at the same time every day.
- Use bed for sleeping only. Avoid reading, watching TV in bed.
- If you do not fall asleep within 20 to 30 minutes of retiring to bed, get up, leave the room and do something which may make you tired. When you feel sleepy try again. Do not lie in bed for more that 30 minutes without sleeping.
- Avoid stimulants (coffee, cigarettes) and avoid alcohol after 4pm.
- You may have to eliminate coffee and cigarettes completely.
- Avoid eating late in the evening.
- Exercise regularly. A brisk walk for 30 to 60 minutes each day is excellent.
- Be careful not to exercise too late in the evening.
- Improve the sleep environment. Darken the room. Ask people to consider your sleep needs. Try earplugs or a blindfold.
- Count sheep? NO! Try not to concentrate on specific problems or worry. For some people, reading can clear their mind. Remember if you can't sleep, get up and leave the room.
- Perform relaxation breathing exercises, see page 165.

Sleeping pills

Most sleeping pills can be addictive or you can become dependent upon them. Studies show that the ability of these drugs to help you sleep wears off after about 2 weeks of regular use, and after this time, people are dependent on them. These medications may also change the pattern of sleep and reduce the length of time we spend in the restorative sleep pattern. These medications may also result in memory problems, concentration difficulties and residual daytime sleepiness. Despite all these problems, you should discuss these sleep medications with your doctor. A short-term trial of one of these drugs may break your insomnia cycle and allow you to sleep better again without medication.

Over-the-counter sleep aids should be avoided. These medications are not designed specifically to help sleep, but commonly cause people to be drowsy. Occasionally, they have a reverse effect. We recommend you discuss medications for sleep with your doctor.

Alcohol is not a sleep aid and should be avoided as therapy for insomnia.

Memory Problems and Dementia

SUMMARY: Having a problem remembering someone's name, an address or how much salt to add to the recipe is annoying. Forgetting the names of your children, your own address or how old you are is a serious problem. Dementia is a brain illness which makes it hard for a person to remember recent events and affects communication and learning. Eventually the person with dementia will be unable to care for themselves. Having some reduction in memory is not unexpected with advancing age; however, age alone should not be the explanation for an inability to remember recent events. Many people recognize that they are having memory problems and become frustrated when they can't remember things. Progressive difficulty with memory and subsequent confusion, disorientation and emotional outbursts may result in family disruption, accidents and even injury to the individual.

Possible symptoms or signs of serious memory problems:

▶ loss of recent memory
▶ problems with language
▶ disorientation of place or time
▶ poor decisions on dress, activity, money
▶ getting lost easily
▶ forgetting important events
▶ inappropriate angry outbursts
▶ blaming others for moving things
▶ leaving tasks uncompleted
▶ asking the same question repeatedly
▶ socially withdrawn, not interested

Memory Problems and Dementia

START HERE

MEMORY PROBLEMS

Are you:
- forgetting how to do things you have done many times?
- having trouble learning new things?
- repeating the same story during the same conversation?
- having trouble making decisions?
- forgetting what you have done today?

YES ▶ You Should See Your Doctor

NO

Does your family:
- notice you becoming disinterested in activities you used to do?
- notice you are having a problem with conversations?
- think your memory problem is affecting your daily life?

YES ▶ You Should See Your Doctor

NO

- Do you have trouble remembering the name of someone you just met?
- Do you have problems finding a word you know you know?
- Are you concerned because your family says that your memory is poor?

YES

You probably have normal memory changes.
See HOME SUGGESTIONS on next page.
If you are concerned talk to your doctor.

Memory Problems and Dementia

▶ HOME SUGGESTIONS

To improve your memory:

1   Make lists. It is not a weakness to use a list for shopping, chores or activities. If you want to be really modern, buy a PDA and use an electronic list.

2   Follow a routine. It is always easier to remember what comes next when you do it the same way every time.

3   Try to make associations to remember things. Addresses may be easier to remember when you associate the location with a local landmark.

4   Keep a detailed calendar of upcoming events.

5   Always put your keys, wallet or other important items in the same place.

6   When you meet someone new, repeat their name a couple of times in the conversation to secure that you have remembered it.

7   Finding words you know may come easier when you run through the ABCs. Try it.

8   Keep your mind busy. Don't spend your time watching TV. Word puzzles, crosswords, number puzzles, card games and reading all take much more concentration and mental energy. If you don't use it you'll lose it.

9   A couple of simple tests may help you determine if further evaluation is necessary:

Ask the person with memory problems to remember three objects. Have them repeat the objects immediately for you, then ask again in 5 minutes. In the meantime ask them to draw a clock and the time ten to two. Don't offer anything but a blank page and a pencil. If they can make a normal clock and remember two or three of the objects there is little to worry about. If the clock is not done well and objects cannot be remembered then see your doctor for further evaluation.

General Information

GENERAL INFORMATION

General information

Cold and Allergy Medicines

The stuffy nose and runny red eyes caused by allergies can feel the same as a cold, but they are different. Many non-prescription medicines available at your drug store combine drugs aimed at both colds and allergies in order to be all things to all people. Often these medicines are combined in such a way as to give you lower doses of these medicines than if you were buying them separately. You can, however, buy non-prescription or over-the-counter medicines which are either purely decongestants or antihistamines.

Different people respond in different ways to certain medications or combinations of medications. This may depend upon the cause of your problem, but also upon how each of us reacts to a particular medicine. Some people will find that a certain cold or allergy medication works better for them; as a result, finding the right medicine for you may require some trial and error.

Medicine packaging doesn't always tell you whether the ingredients are antihistamines or decongestants. Instead they give you the chemical names which are difficult to pronounce or remember. Do not be afraid to ask your pharmacist for help; they can be a helpful source of information.

TAKE THIS BOOK WITH YOU WHEN YOU GO SHOPPING FOR COLD OR ALLERGY MEDICATION.

All about Decongestants

Decongestants are medicines which reduce the swelling and dry up the lining of the nasal passages. These medicines are usually taken as a tablet by mouth or as a nasal spray. Decongestants have difficult-to-remember names such as ephedrine, phenylephrine, phenylpropanolamine, pseudoephedrine, and sprays may contain xylometazoline or oxymetazoline. Many of these drugs are similar to adrenaline, a natural substance produced by your body. These medicines may be dangerous for people with serious heart disease or poorly controlled high blood pressure. They can speed up the heart rate and increase blood pressure. Those suffering with asthma should use these medications with caution.

Decongestants are frequently combined with an antihistamine and pain or fever medication like acetaminophen or ibuprofen. Decongestant medicines can be very helpful in relieving some of the symptoms of a cold or sinus congestion. They may also reduce the runny nose of an allergic reaction, but will not stop the allergic reaction like an antihistamine can. Routine use of nasal sprays may actually result in an increased runny nose. Nasal sprays should not be used on a regular or prolonged basis—we recommend a maximum of 3 days.

Some people have extremely uncomfortable eyes during allergic reactions. There are eye drop medications which contain decongestants (naphazoline, xylometazoline) which will help reduce redness. They may also contain weak antihistamines (antazoline or pheniramine). Commonly purchased products include **Visine** and **Vasocon**.

Adults will find that some trial and error may be necessary to find a decongestant, an antihistamine, or combination medications which will give them good relief from cold or allergy symptoms without causing unwanted side-effects. Remember that combination medications, despite the fact they try to be all things to all people, may not be your best choice for all cold symptoms or allergic reactions. Some people will be better off using a pure antihistamine or decongestant medication.

We find that children benefit most from cold medications taken at night, and frequently do not need medicine during the day. The combination of a sedating antihistamine with a decongestant may therefore be useful when taken at night. We suggest a combination medicine like **Dimetapp**.

We recommend that pain medication be taken in pure form and given in the appropriate dose for weight (see page 58).

For children under two years of age we recommend infant preparations. These are more concentrated and therefore require less volume to get a proper dose. Read the label carefully and ask your pharmacist for advice. Watch all children for the development of unwanted hyperactivity with antihistamines. If this does occur, buy products which only contain a decongestant.

All about Antihistamines

Antihistamines are medications which reduce the effect of histamine. Histamine is what causes the runny, red and itchy eyes, runny nose, swollen throat and rashes of allergies. If you take an antihistamine early in your allergic response you can make your reaction less severe. If you take the antihistamine before the reaction starts you may avoid the allergic reaction altogether. Almost all antihistamines are available without a prescription. Please ask your pharmacist.

Antihistamines can be divided into two main groups:

1   those which can make you sleepy (sedating), and

2   those which do not make you sleepy (non-sedating). The first group may well give you a stronger antihistamine effect in an emergency and may work well for skin reactions. These are also helpful when sleeping well is important. (In fact most over-the-counter sleeping pills contain antihistamines as their main ingredient.) Antihistamines are sold in many forms: tablets, nasal spray, eyedrops and lotions. Some will last all day, others have to be taken as often as every 4 hours. The shorter acting medications may be more useful for emergency use. Diphenhydramine (**Benadryl**) is the drug of first choice of many doctors for severe allergic reactions. An eye drop commonly used to prevent allergic reactions is **Opticrom**.

The antihistamines which may cause sedation include diphenhydramine (**Benadryl**), brompheniramine (**Dimetane**), chlorpheniramine (**Chlor-Tripolon**) and clemastine (**Tavist**) to name only a few. They are also available in combination medications, usually with a decongestant and sometimes with something to reduce a cough. They also come with pain and fever medicines like acetaminophen and ibuprofen. In combination with other cold therapy an antihistamine can help give you a much needed sleep. A word of caution: some people may have an opposite reaction and experience an increase in activity and alertness. Children may be described as becoming "hyper". This can happen with any antihistamine.

The non-sedating ("no sleepiness") antihistamine group includes: Astemizole (**Hismanal**), loratadine (**Claritin**) and fexofenadine (**Allegra**). These non-sedating antihistamines are better choices for regular daily use during the allergy season. They help prevent symptoms without making you sleepy. Astemizole may take up to 3 or 4 days to work when taken regularly. Loratadine and terfenadine will work faster. Astemizole (**Hismanal**) has been found to have **potentially serious side-effects** if taken with the antibiotics erythromycin or clarithromycin (**Biaxin**), the antifungal preparation ketoconazole, or the stomach medication, cisapride (**Prepulsid**).

How and When to Use Antibiotics

Infections often result from an exposure to bacteria, viruses or parasites. Many common health problems develop from viral infections. These include the common cold, the flu and gastroenteritis. There is no specific therapy for viral infections and they usually clear up after a few days without any special therapy.

Antibiotics are drugs which are useful in treating people with bacterial infections. Bacterial infections are commonly found in the lung, urine, sinuses, throat, ears and skin. Antibiotics can help slow down or stop the growth of bacteria so that the body's own defences can fight the infection. When you are given a prescription for an antibiotic you will notice that it is given for a certain number of days. It is very important to take the entire prescriptions as instructed on the label. If you only take the medicine for a couple of days and the infection is not completely cleared, it can come back and cause more trouble.

Antibiotics may not kill all bacteria. Some attack a specific kind of bacteria, while others may be able to kill a larger group of bacteria. Your doctor tries to choose an antibiotic medicine which is specific to the bacteria causing your illness. In this way the medicine is not helping to make other bacteria resistant or immune to the drug's effects. For this reason, it is very important to take antibiotics only when we really need them. The flowcharts in this book will help you decide when your illness requires a doctor's attention and possible antibiotic therapy.

Antibiotics can often cause stomach upset or bowel changes. Diarrhea is the most common side-effect of these medicines. If your diarrhea is severe or contains blood, you should contact your doctor or go to the hospital.

Another caution: Some antibiotics can become toxic (poisonous) or weakened if stored for a long time. Unfinished or old medications should be thrown out. If you have a large quantity to throw out, your pharmacist can help. Never give a medicine prescribed for you to someone else.

All About Pain and Fever Medications

Most people are familiar with **Aspirin** and **Tylenol**. These are the brand names of the very common medications ASA (acetylsalicylic acid) and acetaminophen. These medications are used to treat pain and fever. ASA, but not acetaminophen, can also relieve inflammation (swelling, heat or redness).

One of the new medications you can buy at your pharmacy without a prescription is ibuprofen (**Advil**, **Motrin** and others). This medication belongs to the same family of medications to which ASA belongs. These are Nonsteroidal Anti-Inflammatory Drugs or, as they are sometimes called, NSAIDs. These medicines can relieve pain, lower a fever, and also reduce inflammation. You might think that these medicines are the best overall for they can be used for both pain and inflammation. Unfortunately they can cause stomach ulcers and kidney problems in some people. Sometimes they upset your stomach if not taken with food.

ASA should not be given to people under the age of 20 when they have a viral illness because of a liver disease called Reye's Syndrome which may be caused by taking ASA during influenza infections and the chicken pox. ASA, which stands for acetylsalicylic acid, is from a drug group called salicylates. Another member of this group of medicines is bismuth subsalicylate (**Peptobismol**). We recommend that you do not give these medicines to those under 20 years of age.

Ibuprofen (**Advil**, **Motrin** and others), an NSAID as described above, does not carry the same risk of causing Reye's Syndrome. It can be used alone or occasionally along with acetaminophen in those whose pain and fever does not respond well to acetominophen. Ibuprofen may also relieve discomfort for a longer time (6 to 8 hours versus 4 to 6 hours for acetaminophen). Ibuprofen is also sold in children's strength. Acetaminophen remains the first choice for pain and fever in children. We feel acetaminophen has the best overall safety profile.

You may have heard people say that one or other of these medications works better for their pain. Although this may have been the case, often the problem in controlling pain is that the appropriate dose of the medicine has not been taken. This is especially true in treating children's illnesses. The instructions on the package usually suggests dosages based on age and as a result only the lightest people in an age group get the right dose. You can manage pain better if you take the correct dosage based on your weight. We have created an acetaminophen dosage schedule to make this easier (see page 58). Adults require between 600 and 1000 mg of acetaminophen every 4 hours to relieve pain.

Regular acetaminophen tablets contain 325mg and the extra strength tablets contain 500mg. Serious pain will require 2 to 3 regular tablets or 2 extra strength tablets. You should look carefully at the bottles and price them by the number of effective doses available in the bottle. Ibuprofen dosage should be individualized at 10mg per kg body weight every 6 to 8 hours. Adults can take up to 800mg every 8 hours, but should use the lowest dose that is effective.

There are several pain medications which add caffeine to ASA. This combination can help to improve the effectiveness of the ASA, but is not necessary in most situations. The caffeine content is equivalent to about a half cup of coffee.

Sometimes a narcotic-type medication is added to ASA or acetaminophen to improve the pain relieving effect. Usually codeine is added. By adding 8 mg of codeine to the regular tablets they can produce a medicine which is stronger but still available without a prescription. You will have to ask your pharmacist for this type of medication.

REMEMBER: When you are using a medicine for relieving pain or for controlling a fever, you will be most successful if you give the medicine at regular intervals. If you wait until the pain is really bad or until the fever has crept really high again, it will take longer to get under control. See page 58 for acetaminophen dosage.

Handwashing

Many preventable infections are passed between people by physical contact. Germs of many kinds can remain active on skin, door handles, handrails and other objects for several hours. Since we cannot help contacting objects that others have touched, we need to reduce the transfer of infection by cleansing our hands of these germs.

Handwashing is your best defence against infection. Be sure to wash with soap and running warm water for at least 45 seconds—most people only wash their hands for 5 to 10 seconds.

Today we have available alcohol-based hand sanitizers that kill bacteria and viruses on skin. These sanitizers can irritate some people's skin, but can be purchased with added hand lotion to help protect your skin.

We recommend that you use soap and water to wash away obvious dirt. To better protect yourself and your family from infection and before food preparation you should follow handwashing with an alcohol-based hand sanitizer. In addition, you can use a hand lotion once or twice a day to help keep your skin healthy.

SARS, Bird Flu, West Nile Virus and other Viral Infections

Some viruses can cause infections of the lung called pneumonia including influenza, the SARS virus and bird flu virus. These viruses can be transmitted through inhalation of the droplets in a cough from an infected person. These droplets can be picked up by others by touching objects which have been coughed on. Your best defense from any infection is to make sure that you wash your hands and use hand sanitizers as outlined in the **HANDWASHING** section of this book.

If you develop a respiratory illness with fever, it is prudent not to expose people to your illness. Stay home from work and follow good handwashing techniques. Avoid using the same towels, cloths or utensils as others without proper cleaning. Using a mask will reduce the spread of droplets to your care givers—hospital workers use special N95 masks that filter very small particles, but most droplet spread can be prevented by using a simple operating room-type mask.

If you are not too sick, you may be able to recover well at home. You will remain infectious to others for up to 10 days after you have become well yourself, so we recommend that you remain away from work for 10 days after you have recovered.

If your symptoms become severe or if you have difficulty breathing, eating or managing at home, you should go to hospital with your mask on. You will likely be isolated until a diagnosis can be made.

Vaccination for the flu each fall is still your best bet for prevention. Many people have heard of the medication **Tamiflu**, which is a drug that was initially marketed to treat the common respiratory flu. **Tamiflu** may also be effective in reducing the symptoms and length of illness from bird flu, though this has not been proved. We do not recommend you get a supply of Tamiflu at this time.

Until recently, the western world has not had to deal with mosquito-transmitted diseases. We have all heard of malaria, but most western doctors have never seen a case of it. **West Nile disease** is a new mosquito-transmitted infection. The virus is actually fatal to birds but should not be confused with bird flu. After a bird is infected, mosquitoes may pick up the infection from the bird and transmit it to humans. Generally, the infection is annoying but not fatal to humans. It may, however, be more severe in the elderly or those who are already ill. If you are infected and recover, you will become immune to further infection. A vaccination for West Nile is not yet available, and the best way to prevent infection is to protect yourself from insect bites.

Mosquito and insect bite prevention

The best prevention for insect bites is avoidance. Avoid outdoor activity at dusk. To prevent insect bites, cover up by wearing long pants and shirts with long sleeves or a bug jacket. Using insect repellant containing DEET will reduce bites from mosquitoes and other biting insects. DEET solutions are available in 10-30% strengths. Be aware that higher percentage solutions are not "stronger" nor do they do repel better. A higher DEET percentage means that you can wait longer before reapplying more repellant. If you use a 10% solution, you may have to reapply every two hours.

You can also reduce the potential for mosquito bites by preparing your clothes and your tent in advance. Apply a 0.25% or 0.5% solution of PERMETHRIN (**NIX**)

INFORMATION

to clothing or other fabrics. Spray the material so that it is wet then let it dry. **This substance is not a bug repellant and should not be applied to the skin.** It is the same product that is used to treat head lice, and works by causing damage to the mosquito's nervous system.

The combination of PERMETHRIN prepared clothing and camping equipment and the application of DEET to exposed skin is an excellent way of reducing your risk of insect bites while enjoying the great outdoors.

Immunization

There is likely nothing we have done medically as a society that has saved as many lives as immunization. Some people have lost both their fear of some serious illnesses and their respect for the power of the vaccination because we rarely see these dangerous conditions and their complications anymore.

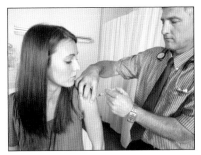

Safety of vaccines

There is a segment of the population that believes that vaccinations are more dangerous than the conditions they prevent. These individuals put their children at risk by avoiding vaccination based on unproven concerns about vaccination safety. Immunization is still the best way to protect children and adults from many serious diseases.

Vaccines are extremely safe, with serious side-effects rare and severe allergic reactions occurring less than one in a million. Minor side-effects, such as redness, swelling or low fever, are not unusual but last only a short time. It is vital to remember that the risk of the disease is much greater than risks associated with the vaccine.

Are immunizations still needed?

When immunization levels in a population drop, these diseases start to reappear because we have not eliminated them, just protected ourselves from them at a point in time. The ideal goal is to have the entire population immunized which may result in the elimination of these diseases that have killed so many in the past. Remember that smallpox was once a deadly illness which was eliminated by a universal vaccination program.

How do vaccines work? (Are they "unnatural?")

Immunization works very simply. The body is exposed to either a part of an infectious agent (bacteria or virus) or a de-activated agent in a small dose. This stimulates an immune response so that if you are exposed to the real infection, your body is ready with an already prepared immune response. In this way, our immune system works "naturally" to protect us from re-infection by the same virus or bacteria. So while some people argue that immunization is not "natural", it is no more unnatural than getting the disease itself.

To illustrate this concept, we can look at the chickenpox virus. In the past, almost all children caught chickenpox. Children and adults can be exposed to the infection many times, but still only get chickenpox once. Having once had the illness, the immune system is ready for it a second time with a protective response. It is this protective immune response that is stimulated by immunization. We are using our immune system to be preventive rather than only using it to react to illness. So, in fact, immunizations do not weaken our immune system, rather immunization uses the immune system to our advantage.

Adult immunization

If you received your childhood series of immunizations, you may still need the following;

- dTap (diptheria, tetanus and pertusis-whooping cough): You need a booster every 10 years.
- Hepatitis B: Anyone who is at risk of blood or body fluid contact should be immunized. This is a series of three shots.
- Flu shot: This is an annual shot that is especially important for the elderly and those with serious medical conditions, but will protect individuals of any age.
- Pneumococcus (pneumonia shot): This is a one-time vaccine to prevent the most common cause of bacterial pneumonia. This does not, however, protect from all forms of pneumonia.

Immunization for international travellers

Travellers should consider being vaccinated for Hepatitis A. Other vaccinations may be required, depending on the location visited.

If you are planning to travel outside the country, please check with the website below or talk to your doctor six months before you plan to leave to find out what immunizations are required and/or recommended for your destination.

Make sure your children's immunizations, as well as yours, are up-to-date.

For reliable information on immunization visit:
Public Health Agency of Canada www.phac-aspc.gc.ca
Health Canada www.hc-sc-gc.ca

Dieting and Weight Loss

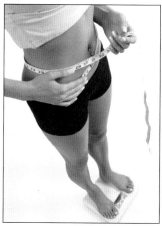

Obesity increases the risk of many diseases, including diabetes, high blood pressure, heart attack, stroke and joint problems. Although it generally takes many years to become overweight, when people want to lose weight, they want to do so quickly, easily and cheaply. Unfortunately, a magical weight loss therapy does not exist.

Fad diets may result in some short-term weight loss, but are usually so difficult to continue that, unless you replace your less healthy habits with better overall diet habits, your weight will increase again. As a general rule, if a diet requires unusual food choices or patterns of eating, or complicated preparation and appears too difficult to sustain, you are unlikely to achieve long-term weight loss. Some diets, however, can kick-start your weight loss which can then be maintained if other lifestyle and healthy eating habits are adopted.

People eat food for energy. We use energy to live, breathe and undertake physical work. The more active you are, the more calories you burn. If you become less active, the extra calories are stored as fat. Once we have a large reserve of energy stored as fat in our bodies, we have to be prepared to take time to lose weight even if we starve ourselves. This is because our bodies will try to defend themselves from starvation. When you drastically reduce your food intake, your metabolism will slow down to protect your body from starving.

The most successful way to lose weight is to combine a reasonable reduction in food intake with an increase in regular exercise, and to be patient. Some weight loss diets are based on reducing the number of calories you eat every day to slowly reduce the storage fat. Others are designed to fool your body into preferentially burning the fat you have previously stored.

Goals of weight loss

We measure healthy weight by calculating your Body Mass Index (BMI) which compares your weight to your height.

$$\textbf{Body Mass Index (BMI)} = \frac{\text{Weight in Kilograms}}{(\text{Height in meters})^2}$$

Conversion (1 kg is 2.2 pounds, 1 inch = 2.5cm)

So a 5'11" man who weighs 200lbs would have a BMI of $\dfrac{90.9\text{kg}}{(1.775\text{m})^2} = 28.85$ kg/m2

A BMI of 25 to 29 suggests you are overweight and a BMI of greater than 30 is considered obesity. A higher BMI may not always mean you have too much fat, however, because muscle weighs more than fat—if you are well muscled, you may have a higher BMI but not be fat.

The Canadian Task Force on Preventive Health recommends weight loss for anyone with a BMI greater than 27 **and at least one obesity-related disease**. If you lose as little as 5-10% of your weight, you will reduce your risks of heart disease and stroke.

Another way to decide if you have too much fat is to consider your body type. Pear-shaped people have fat at their hips and thighs. Apple-shaped people are fatter in the middle. Apple-shaped people are at higher risk of stroke, heart disease and diabetes. A waist measurement for men of over 40in (102cm) measured at the belly button or greater than 35in (88cm) for women measured half way between the ribs and the hips means an increased risk of heart disease, stroke and diabetes. These people should lose weight. For more information visit the Heart and Stroke Foundation web site at **www.heartandstroke.ca**.

Types of diets

Generally there are four types of diets:

- **Low Calorie**
- **Very Low Calorie**
- **Low Carbohydrate**
- **Very Low Fat**

Conversion	
Calorie(cal)	Kilojoule(kj)
1	4.2
10	42
100	420
1000	4200

Although diets have different names and people will have different theories as to how they work, they all generally tend to reduce the amount of food people eat.

Fat is very high in calories. Every gram of fat has 9 calories, while every gram of protein or carbohydrate has about 4 calories. This means that for every gram of fat you eat, you get twice the number of calories of a similar amount of protein or carbohydrate. It would appear on the surface then that lowering your fat intake will result in a significant reduction in the intake of food energy and result in weight loss.

The common **low calorie** diets use this information to design a diet that is lower in fat (less than 30% of total calories consumed) and relatively higher in carbohydrates (55-60% of calories) to reduce your overall calorie intake. If these diets contain increased amounts of fibre (which fills you up), you can satisfy your hunger and reduce your overall intake of food. You must also avoid simple sugars and eat instead the complex carbohydrates found in fruits and vegetables. **Low calorie** diets usually recommend a daily calorie reduction of between 500-1000 calories (2100-4200kj) per day or a total intake of between 1000 and 1400 calories (4200-5880kj) per day.

Low calorie diets can reduce body weight by about 8% over 3 to 12 months. Usually only half of the initial weight loss is maintained over the next three or four years. These same diets have been shown to reduce waist circumference by up to 9.5cm. To truly reduce the risk of heart disease with **low calorie** diets, you must also adopt a regular exercise program.

Very low calorie diets contain only 800 calories (3360kj) per day. This kind of diet usually requires a special food formula to supply the proper amount of protein to prevent starvation. These diets are usually only used by those with a BMI over 30 who face significant health risks and who have failed previous weight loss attempts. These diets can result in a 20kg (44lbs) weight loss within 16 weeks. Side-effects of these diets may include gallstone formation, loss of muscle mass and gout. If the protein intake in these very **low calorie diets** is not adequate, there have been cases of sudden death.

The **low carbohydrate** diet was initially introduced as the Atkins diet in the 1970s but has been modified and copied by many authors in different forms. All low carbohydrate diets reduce the amount of carbohydrates in the diet to less than 10% of all calories or about 30g of carbohydrate per day. This tends to reduce the total calorie intake to 1300 cal or 5460kj per day through the relative reduction in appetite from eating larger amounts of protein or fat, as well as the restricted food choices.

Some theorize that this diet makes the body use fat stores to generate energy because the restriction of carbohydrates severely limits the body's access to easy energy. Many swear by this diet due to its association with early rapid weight loss. Some of this may be due to a reduction in total body water (1 litre weighs 1kg) caused by a total reduction in carbohydrate stores. Initially some experts suggested that these diets might cause adverse changes to cholesterol levels and may cause kidney damage, but these problems have not been demonstrated in studies looking at these diets over the first year.

Very low fat diets recommend that you take only 10-15% of your total calorie intake from fat. These diets were introduced to prevent or reduce heart disease, and were popularized by Dr. Ornish. The Ornish diet trial used a vegetarian diet with 10% of calories from fat, smoking cessation, stress management and aerobic exercise to obtain 10.9kg weight loss in year one. These patients were not taking cholesterol-reducing medications, but still showed a reduction of coronary artery disease by 4.5% in year 1 and 7.9% in year 5. In comparison, patients on a regular diet showed a deterioration of heart disease by 5.4% in year 1 and 27.7% in year 5.

Despite these results, the American Heart Association warns against **very low fat** diets because the increased carbohydrate intake may increase the body's triglyceride fat levels, which may be harmful and the very large amount of fibre (more than twice the recommended level) may reduce the absorption of calcium, iron and zinc by your body, and may increase symptoms of abdominal fullness and bloating.

RECOMMENDATIONS

Although many have found that pushing away from the table is difficult, the best way to reduce weight is to combine a sensible reduction in total food intake with an increase in exercise. Weight loss may occur slowly but will be sustainable. Maintaining a diet that is very restrictive or unpalatable is very difficult, and those who look for a quick fix will find that they fall back on old habits quickly and gain the weight back.

A better approach is to learn to eat better. Some easy calorie reductions include adding less sugar to cereals, using only jam instead of butter and jam on toast, cutting out mayonnaise, and cutting alcohol intake in half.

You don't have to buy a new machine in order to exercise. You can get the exercise you need from a daily 30-minute brisk walk. Try taking the walk before you eat—it may help curb your appetite.

Be wary of magical solutions. If you do follow a low carbohydrate or low fat diet to jumpstart your weight loss, you should switch to a more moderate approach for long-term weight loss maintenance.

Many of us need a plan. There are many organizations that recommend moderate calorie reduction without the need for dramatic changes—look at Canada's Food Guide at **www.hc-sc.gc.ca**, the Canadian Diabetes Association meal planner at **www.diabetes.ca** or the Heart and Stroke Foundation at **www.heartandstroke.ca** for examples.

Exercise

Few things improve health and your sense of well-being as much as regular exercise. Exercise helps you feel good physically and feel good about yourself emotionally. For many, exercise becomes a treasured and guarded part of their day.

Benefits of regular exercise

- Regular exercise reduces the risk of heart disease, stroke, high blood pressure, obesity and osteoporosis.
- Regular exercise helps to control weight by burning calories, increasing your metabolic rate and surpressing appetite.
- Getting regular exercise now increases the chances that you will be a lifelong exerciser.
- Regular exercise reduces stress and decreases anxiety.
- Regular exercise helps you sleep more soundly.
- Regular exercise strengthens muscles and helps keep joints flexible.
- Regular exercise can increase energy levels.
- Regular exercisers are often less prone to depression.
- People who exercise feel better about themselves.

How do I get started?

If you have been inactive for some time, you will need to start your exercise program slowly and gradually increase the frequency and/or the length of your sessions. You can also begin by exercising every second day rather than every day. A little pain and soreness are perfectly normal when your muscles are not accustomed to exercise, but a good rule of thumb is that if you feel significant pain, stiffness or fatigue the day after you exercise, you have done too much and need to temporarily cut back. It is vitally important that you realize that exercise may not be fun and invigorating for the first six to eight weeks of your program, but once you have built up to a certain level of fitness, you will begin to enjoy what you are doing. Be patient, push on and don't quit in the early stages. Think long term!

Ensure your success

Set realistic goals. Remember that any exercise is better than doing nothing. By setting initial goals that are too high you increase your chances of feeling like a failure. Pushing too hard too soon may cause pain and increases the chance you will stop regular exercise.

Select the right type of exercise. If you enjoy what you are doing then you are more likely to continue for the longer term. Some people find it beneficial to change activities from day to day, while others like to concentrate on just one type.

Find someone who you enjoy being with and who shares the same goals as you. Partners can be motivating and make us accountable.

Schedule your exercise. People who leave exercise unscheduled and try to squeeze it in when they have a chance rarely reach their goals. Put it on the calendar.

Keep a logbook that records your exercise, distances, and times etc. You will be encouraged by your progress when you look back.

Don't push it when it hurts. Pain is not productive and is your body trying to tell you something.

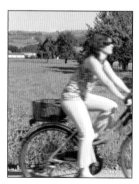

What is exercise?

Many people feel that they do not need to exercise because they are active every day. They believe that gardening, walking at work or working around the house are ways of getting a lot of exercise. However, you can be very active and very tired at the end of the day, yet have done very little exercise. Often the activity that we do is of a "stop and start" nature and is not continuous. Real exercise requires a prolonged increase in heart rate. This only occurs with continuous exercise. The goal of a heart healthy exercise program is a continuous 30 to 40-minute daily workout.

How much should I exercise?

Start slowly. Beginning too aggressively increases the likelihood of quitting. The goal is to exercise 30 to 40 minutes daily. If you have been inactive, begin with easier workouts every second day and slowly increase the frequency. Successful exercisers plan and schedule their daily exercise.

Aerobic exercise and target heart rate

Aerobic exercise uses your large muscle groups (arms, chest, shoulders and especially the legs) in a continuous workout that does not result in rapid shortness of breath and the need to stop. This is great for the health of your heart and lungs. One of the tools that some people use is the target heart rate (THR). Take your pulse for 15 seconds and multiply by four to get your heart rate in beats per minute. Using the chart, you can find the heart rate that is in your "aerobic" range. For a beginner, aim for a heart rate at the 60% level. As you increase your fitness, move towards the 85% level. Do not try and take your pulse while you are exercising. Instead, stop briefly and take your pulse and then adjust the intensity of your exercise.

Exercise Target Heart Rate Chart

Individuals taking medications which may govern or slow heart rates should discuss these targets with their doctor.

AGE	LOW FITNESS	SOME FITNESS	AVERAGE FITNESS	ABOVE AVEAGE FITNESS
30	76-95	95-114	114-152	133-171
35	74-93	93-111	111-148	130-167
40	72-90	90-108	108-144	126-162
45	70-88	88-105	105-140	122-158
50	68-85	85-102	102-136	119-153
55	66-83	83-99	96-132	112-144
60	64-80	80-96	96-178	112-144
65	62-78	78-93	93-124	109-140
70	60-75	75-90	90-120	105-135
75	58-73	73-87	87-116	102-131
80	56-70	70-84	84-112	98-126

Exercise, arthritis and osteoporosis

Regular exercise is a key component of a comprehensive program to treat or prevent osteoporosis (weak or brittle bones). To achieve the benefits of exercise for your bones, you need to find exercises that require you to support your weight on your feet. Examples include walking, running, skating and skiing.

Swimming is great exercise. With the water supporting your weight, your joints do not suffer the same strain as from other exercise. Swimming and other water sports are better choices for those with arthritis or other joint problems which limit walking or running. Riding a bike or exercise cycle can be an excellent choice for those with painful hips, knees or ankles. Keeping your joints active, flexible and strong is good for everyone with arthritis.

Exercise

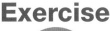

READY TO START EXERCISING

- Have you been very inactive for many years?
- Are you over age 60?
- Do you have heart disease, lung disease or diabetes?
- Are you pregnant?
- Do you have other chronic health problems?
- Are you grossly overweight or a long-time smoker?

YES ▶ **You Should See Your Doctor**

NO

- Have you ever passed out during exercise? **YES** ▶ **You Should See Your Doctor**

NO

When you exercise do you get;
- Chest pain or tightness?
- Are you short of breath with minimal exercise?
- Significant bone, joint, or muscle pain?
- Light-headed or dizzy?

YES ▶ **You Should See Your Doctor**

NO

Enjoy starting to exercise.

Smoking

Smoking has both immediate and long-term consequences for your health. Most smokers begin at a young age, often to fit in, and the immediate effects of bad breath and smelly clothes are not considered important. Smoking may seem painless at the time and for this reason many people do not feel a need to quit—it is easy to smoke when the long-term consequences are a long way off. Stopping smoking at any time reduces the long-term risks and consequences: It is never too late to butt out.

Smoking increases the risk of*:

- Heart disease
- Stroke
- Circulation problems
- High blood pressure
- Lung cancer
- High cholesterol
- Cancer of the mouth, throat and larynx (voice box)
- Cancer of the pancreas

- Cancer of the kidney and bladder
- Chronic bronchitis
- Emphysema
- Pneumonia
- Common colds
- Stomach ulcers
- Inflammatory bowel disease
- Tooth decay
- Gum disease
- Osteoporosis
- Sleep problems
- Cataracts
- Thyroid disease
- Skin wrinkles (premature aging)
- Your children becoming smokers (the risk doubles)

For females, smoking also increases the risks of:

- Cancer of the cervix
- Menstrual problems
- Fertility problems
- Miscarriage

For males, smoking increases the risk of:

- Erectile dysfunction
- Fertility problems

From Health Canada 2007.

Second-hand smoke

Two-thirds of the smoke from a cigarette goes straight into the air and not into the smoker's lungs. Regular exposure to second-hand smoke increases the possibility of lung disease by 25% and heart disease by 10%. Children actually absorb more of the toxins from the smoke than adults do. Electronic air exchange systems do not eliminate second-hand smoke—smoking in one part of the house or opening a window does not make the house safe.

HOME SUGGESTIONS

1   It is vital that you set a quit date which can be two, four or six weeks away—not tomorrow unless you are ready. We advise you to set your quit date well in advance so you have time to prepare. Tell other people that you are going to quit so that you feel obligated to keep the date firm. Try to cut down in advance to make the final step easier. You must prepare yourself mentally for what may be a hard battle.

2   Build support. Look to friends and family for their encouragement. Tell them your quit date and how they might help you. It is very important that you involve your friends who are smokers as they can either make it very difficult for you or be very supportive.

3   Identify the habits or activities that you associate with smoking. Make a list of the regular times and places that you have a cigarette. If you always have a cigarette: with your coffee, in the lunch room with your co-workers or right after dinner, change those activities so that you do not miss the cigarettes as much. When you eliminate the activity that you associate with smoking, you can often avoid the cigarette without much problem. It is helpful to try to figure out why you smoke: Is it for the relaxation, the social interaction or is it just a ritual? If you can identify the reason why you smoke, you can look for other ways to meet that need.

4   Put the money that you would have spent on cigarettes away in a special place or bank account. For many smokers, this can be very motivating as the savings can quickly add up to a nice vacation or other reward.

5   Learn relaxation techniques to help relieve the stress caused by nicotine withdrawal.

6   Join a stop smoking program.

7   Read all the stop smoking material that you can find.

Your doctor can help you with

1   Nicotine replacement gum. Chew a piece of this gum until the craving for a cigarette passes, and then spit it out. Nicotine replacement gum now comes in a better tasting form than previous versions, and no prescription is required.

2   Nicotine patches. There are three strengths of patches: 7 mg, 14 mg and 21 mg. For many people, the 21 mg patch is too strong so we advise that you start with the 14 mg patch. If you need to go stronger, then you will use the 14 mg patches as you taper back down from 21mg. When you have suppressed the cravings for several weeks, you can move to a lower strength. You can stop using the patches when you have had several weeks without cravings while using the 7mg dose.

   Do not smoke while using nicotine patches. Nicotine overdoses may occur. Some people remove the patch to have a cigarette and then put it back on. This is still dangerous as the patch has put a level of nicotine into your blood that does not instantly disappear when you take the patch off. If you simply cannot refrain from smoking, then nicotine patches are not for you. Nicotine patches are available without a prescription.

3   There are two prescription medications that may help some people quit smoking. Talk to your doctor about **Zyban** or **Champix**.

Quitting (tapering vs cold turkey)

Quitting suddenly and all at once is the only way to go for some people. For others, who feel the physical effects of withdrawal strongly, cold turkey can be pretty tough. Quitting smoking means that you must break the habit, as well as beat the physical symptoms of withdrawal. The addiction (your body's craving for nicotine) can have a much stronger hold on some people than others, which is not necessarily related to how much or for how long you have smoked. Because everyone's body is different, tapering off may be a better way quit for some people.

Here are a few tips to increase the chances of a successfully quitting by tapering off:

- Start at a level that is only a couple of cigarettes a day below your usual amount.

- Plan to decrease by a cigarette or two every 7 to 14 days.

- Do not carry more cigarettes than are allowed for the day.

- When you are smoking only one or two cigarettes per day, you are ready to quit.

- Be prepared for a relapse. A stressful day or family crisis may cause you to smoke more. If this happens, don't abandon the plan. Pick things up again the next day and continue to taper off, or if you had successfully quit, become a non-smoker again.

Disease Prevention and Detection

We are all born with specific potentials. Some of us, given the right interest and training, may become exceptional athletes, while others may become gifted scientists.

Unfortunately, this rule also applies to health problems. For some people, exposure to cigarette smoke will cause lung cancer, while others will develop diabetes if they become obese. For many, heart disease is common in their family. Given the right circumstances, we may all be at risk for one ailment or another.

Some diseases are so common in society that it is difficult to determine why a certain person has developed the disorder. Examples of common ailments include heart disease, diabetes, stroke and certain cancers such as lung, colon, breast and prostate.

Through careful study over time, we have been able to determine some of the factors that increase the risk of developing a specific disease. From these studies, we can point to changes in behavior or improved chemical exposure profiles that will reduce the chances of developing a serious condition early in life.

Prevention is difficult and is like trying to win the lottery. If we could predict with accuracy who was going to get lung cancer, we could target those who need to work to prevent it. Unfortunately, we cannot predict these diseases that well. This means that we treat or recommend medication, testing or lifestyle changes for large groups of people, even though only a few will be likely to get the disease.

As an example, let's look at the risk of stroke associated with high blood pressure. High blood pressure increases your risk of having a stroke. We have to treat about 110 people successfully to prevent one stroke. This means that the other 109 people do not really benefit from the treatment. It would be great if we could get a room full of 110 people and get one of them to volunteer to have the stroke. Then we wouldn't have to treat the rest. No volunteers eh?

This example demonstrates how we must apply a screening test, medication treatment or lifestyle change to large populations of people who are all at some increased risk to make the required reduction in risk for the few who will really benefit. We all wear seatbelts, but only a few of us benefit from the seatbelt during an accident each day.

There are two types of prevention measures we take. The first is primary prevention, where we work to prevent the disease before any evidence of it has appeared. Stopping smoking to prevent lung cancer is a good example of primary prevention. We can also try to stop the progress of an illness once it has appeared, which is secondary prevention. Working to reduce a patient's cholesterol levels after they have suffered a heart attack is an example of secondary prevention.

Points to remember

- No one is at zero risk for disease. Some have greater risk than others.
- Prevention means testing, treatment or changes to reduce risk.
- Primary prevention means prevention before the disease begins.
- Secondary prevention means trying to stop the progression of disease.

Heart Disease and Heart Attack

Your heart is a pump. It doesn't get its energy, oxygen and nutrients from the blood that goes through it. Instead, there are small blood vessels that run over the outer surface of the heart that deliver the oxygen and nutrients directly to the muscle.

These small blood vessels may develop narrowings as a result of the deposit of cholesterol in the walls and a reaction of the wall to the deposit of fat. As long as the opening in the artery is greater than 50% of its full size, you will feel nothing. When the narrowings start to get tighter, however, they may reduce the amount of blood that can reach the muscle. If tight enough, you may lack proper oxygen supply to the heart muscle and experience pain or angina when you ask your heart to do more work. This pain may be a tightening, pressure, burning or aching discomfort. It may be felt in the chest, arms, neck or even your back. It may go away when you sit down or stop doing whatever it was that brought on the pain. Occasionally this same symptom may occur when you are at rest or may wake you from sleep.

Heart disease may also present in a different manner. A heart attack occurs when one of these narrowings suddenly changes. These fat deposits can act as volcanoes and suddenly rupture, activating the clotting mechanism of your blood and causing a clot to form across the artery, stopping all blood flow. When all blood flow stops then the muscle area that was being supplied by the artery will begin to die. If the blockage is in a large branch then it will cause a big heart attack. If it is in a smaller branch then the amount of muscle that may die will be less. Once heart muscle dies, it does not grow back.

Although it would be better to prevent heart attacks altogether, we can treat heart attacks if people come to hospital soon enough, and the sooner the better. Remember, with every passing minute some of the heart muscle is dying because of a lack of oxygen. We have special medications that will allow the blood clot to dissolve and return the blood flow and oxygen to the heart muscle. If treated within 4 to 6 hours, there will be a reduction in the ultimate damage suffered.

Detection of heart disease that is slowly developing requires testing which puts the heart at some stress. This means accelerating the heart rate while observing for any evidence of inadequate delivery of oxygen and nutrients to the heart muscle. An exercise stress test and other exercise tests using nuclear medicine may help identify people with significant artery narrowings. An angiogram is the ultimate test for the presence of the narrowings, where dye is injected into the small arteries which is detected by x-ray. The angiogram road map will help cardiologists and cardiac surgeons decide if a patient may benefit from dilating arteries with balloons (angioplasty) or whether they require bypass surgery.

Points to remember

- Artery narrowing reduces blood flow to heart muscle.
- Narrowings usually do not cause symptoms until more than 50% narrowed.
- Blood clots may form at narrowings suddenly.
- Medications can reverse the clotting and stop heart attacks.
- Go to hospital as soon as symptoms develop. Time is heart muscle.
- Exercise testing and nuclear medicine tests may show if narrowings exist.
- Angiogram testing will show where the narrowings are.

Stroke

A stroke refers to the sudden loss of brain function in a specific area. It can occur as a result of a blockage of an artery by a clot, or it may involve a rupture of a brain blood vessel and bleeding within the brain. As with heart disease, some people may have symptoms that spontaneously reverse over several minutes. These are warning episodes and are called TIAs or Transient Ischemic Attacks.

Symptoms of a stroke may include:

- a sudden severe headache
- sudden loss of vision
- sudden loss of muscle control
- sudden loss of balance or loss of feeling to arm, leg or face
- sudden confusion or loss of speech

Unlike a heart attack, there is much less time to try and return normal blood flow to the brain. The window of opportunity is only about three hours, so it is vital to get to the hospital without delay if you or a family member suffers these symptoms. The same clot-dissolving medication used to stop heart attacks can be used on some stroke victims.

Points to remember

- Transient Ischemic Attacks (TIAs) are short reversible episodes of brain dysfunction. These are warnings of a stroke to come.
- Strokes may be reversed with clot-dissolving drugs.
- Some strokes are due to bleeding in the brain.
- Go to hospital immediately if you develop any of the symptoms listed above.

Prevention of Heart Attack and Stroke

It is impossible to know who will develop significant heart disease or stroke. We know some of us have a greater risk of these diseases than others. Unfortunately, even those at low risk can suffer a stroke or heart attack so we must all be ready to seek help if we suffer new symptoms.

We know that artery disease means that narrowings are forming in the arteries that supply your heart, brain, limbs or other organs with blood and oxygen. Anything that may cause these narrowings to increase will bring on symptoms sooner, and risk factors include:

- High blood cholesterol
- Diabetes, which causes blood vessel damage; better diabetic control slows the progression of blood vessel disease
- Obesity, which is a major factor in the development of Type 2 diabetes; controlling weigh reduces diabetes and thus heart disease
- Smoking—the chemicals in cigarette smoke may cause injury to the walls of the blood vessels and accelerate the narrowing process. Stopping smoking reduces the increased risk within a couple of years
- High blood pressure may cause increased stress on blood vessels and the heart itself.

Those with higher blood cholesterol levels tend to make narrowings faster. Reducing cholesterol and triglyceride levels in these people may slow the narrowing process. Diabetics develop blood vessel damage more rapidly than non-diabetics. Better diabetic control slows the progression of blood vessel disease. Obesity is one of the major factors in the development of Type 2 diabetes. Controlling weight gain will result in a reduction of diabetes and thus heart disease. Chemicals in cigarette smoke may cause injury to the walls of blood vessels and accelerate the narrowing process. If you stop smoking, this increased risk resolves within a couple of years. Higher blood pressure may cause increased stress on blood vessels and the heart itself. This may accelerate the narrowing process or result in rupture of small brain blood vessels.

We all know that doing anything to excess is probably not healthy. A healthy lifestyle includes 30 minutes of regular daily exercise; having five or fewer alcoholic drinks per week; and a diet that includes a wide variety of fruits and vegetables and a variety of meat sources, including a regular intake of fish.

Remember we were all born with potentials we may not realize. See your doctor to consider screening tests for your potential increased risk of heart disease or stroke.

Points to remember

- Everyone is at risk of heart attack or stroke, some more than others.
- Risk reduction means reducing the chance that artery narrowing progresses.
- Diabetes and poor blood sugar control accelerate the narrowing of arteries.
- Obesity is the number one cause of Type 2 diabetes.
- Stopping smoking reduces the risk of disease progression in a couple of years.
- A healthy lifestyle includes:
  - 30 minutes of exercise daily
  - a variety of fruits and vegetables daily
  - fish in the diet regularly
  - alcohol in moderation
  - maintaining a healthy weight.
- See your doctor to discuss your risk of heart attack or stroke.

Detection and Prevention of Cancer

No one catches cancer—cancer is a mistake. Many of the cells of your body can divide and create new cells. We make new cells in many organs every day. This activity is under strict control. Controlling this division process is a full time job of your immune system. Unfortunately as we age there is an increasing chance that an error in division may develop. In addition exposure to certain infections, chemicals or irritants may cause cells to be more likely to develop errors. If an error occurs and this division process goes out of control then a cancer can be born. These groups of abnormal cells may damage normal tissue around them. The abnormal cells may get into the lymph or blood systems and spread around the body.

Generally cancer growths or masses (collection of cells without normal structure) grow slowly within the organ where they first started. They sometimes begin to spread elsewhere when they have grown to a certain size. This size can be quite small. A mass as little as one to two centimeters contains billions of cells.

Many of our prevention strategies for cancer depend on our ability to find these cancer growths when they are very small. If we are able to treat the patient by removing the cancer at this small size then there is a chance that the patient may be cured. When the cancers grow larger or have spread to other parts of the body then treatment becomes more difficult and the chance of cure is reduced.

Common cancers

We have all seen the advertisements about the common cancers in society. Lung cancer remains the most common cause of serious cancer and cancer death. In women breast cancer is second by a slim margin over colon cancer. In men colon cancer is the second most common cause of cancer death. Prostate cancer is common but doesn't tend to kill as many men. Skin cancer is the most common cancer but generally is easy to treat. Melanoma, a form of skin cancer which develops from the cells with pigment (colour) is much more dangerous but less common.

Cancer detection

It would be great if there was a single test to find all cancers. This does not exist. Doctors try to find cancers at an early stage to increase the chance of cure. Screening tests are used to find cancers before they cause patients symptoms. The tests used to find these cancers are not perfect, however. The perfect cancer test would be one that is easy to perform, does not cause any discomfort, is inexpensive and finds all the people with the cancer. An even better cancer test would be one that tells us who will develop cancer in the future.

Doctors do pay special attention to people with a strong family history of cancer. Some cancers are more common in families. Genetic testing may offer a method of screening family members for an increased risk. Most new cancers, however, develop in people without a family history.

Average risk people (that means most of us) will have to depend on tests that aim to find the cancer before we know we have it. Screening tests have been created to help find some of the common cancers.

Pap smears have been around for a long time. We know that cervical cancer is associated with an infection by a virus called Human Papilloma Virus (HPV). The testing for HPV and the evaluation of the cervix for early cancer cells may be uncomfortable but may lead to life-saving therapy. No woman should deny herself this test. There is now a vaccination available for HPV; women who get vaccinated reduce their chance of getting cervical cancer.

Although not a perfect test, **Mammograms** can detect early breast cancers and may lead to life-saving surgery and treatment. Until a better test appears women should bear the discomfort of the mammogram and be tested regularly. If you have a family history of breast cancer start screening at age 40. If you are of average risk start at age 50.

A blood test for prostate cancer does exist. This is called the **PSA test**. A single test is not as useful as having an annual test. If the level is rising over time further testing is required to see if a cancer is present. We must remember that prostate cancer is very common and often not significant. About 80% of men over 80 will have prostate cancer that causes them no harm. You should also know that some men with prostate cancer may not have a rising PSA test from year to year.

Colon cancer may cause bleeding into the stool in very small amounts invisible to the naked eye. A test showing blood in the stool may be the first clue that there is a cancer present. Most family doctors will do a **Fecal Occult Blood test (FOBT)** every year or two in people over 50 years of age.

At present there is no strategy for screening for lung cancer. Certainly if you are a smoker you might want to consider a **chest x-ray** on a regular basis. Unfortunately smoking may cause changes to the lung which makes interpretation of the chest x-ray difficult. Regular CAT-scans of the chest may also detect cancer in high risk smokers, but these tests are harder to get, are more expensive and cause increased radiation exposure.

Skin examination is the best way to search for changes of skin cancer. Those with fairer skin and those with previous skin cancers or family members with skin cancer may be at increased risk.

Cancer prevention

True cancer prevention means stopping cancer from ever starting. For some cancers prevention requires a change in behaviour. Sometimes prevention means a special test is required to stop the cancer from starting.

Smoking. Smoking greatly increases your risk of lung cancer as well as many other cancers. Smoking is not the only reason for lung cancer, however, and some people with lung cancer have not been exposed to cigarette smoke. Some smokers get other life-threatening lung disease. Predicting which smokers will get which cancer is impossible. Never smoking or stopping smoking is the only real way to reduce your risk of lung cancer. Stopping smoking may also reduce your risk of many other types of cancer.

Chemical or industrial and environment exposure. As time goes on we learn more and more about exposures to chemicals or hazards of the work place and how this might increase the risk of certain cancers. Asbestos, radon gas and benzene are only a few of the substances that we now try to avoid. Outside workers need to protect themselves from exposure to the sun. Sun exposure clearly increases the risk of skin cancer and the most deadly of these is melanoma. Reducing your exposure to sunlight with clothes and hats in addition to using sun screen with SPF of 30 or more on exposed skin is your best bet.

Diet, vitamins, supplements. We get lots of advice about how to eat and what to avoid. Sometimes the new information contradicts what we were told last year. A simple plan which has always been good advice is to take everything in moderation. We should eat a variety of vegetables. It is reasonable to control our intake of fats and overall calories so as not to become obese. We should avoid eating only beef. Add some fish to your diet. There is little evidence to suggest that taking extra vitamin B, C, E, or others will reduce your risk of cancers. In fact as time goes on we are collecting data that many of these supplement vitamins may well increase your risk of heart disease and other complications. If someone insists that they have the cure for anything ask to see their Nobel Prize. Don't have one? Question the proof of cure or prevention.

True Cancer Prevention. Cervical and colon cancer are truly preventable. The human papilloma virus vaccines will prevent many young women from developing cervical cancer. There is evidence suggesting that most colon cancers develop from a growth in the colon called a polyp. These polyps are common, but if removed before becoming cancerous then cancer can be prevented. To find out if you have polyps you must undergo either an x-ray study called a barium enema, have a CT-scan called CT Colography or have a scope test called colonoscopy. If you are over 50 years of age, you should ask your doctor about colon screening.

High Blood Pressure (Hypertension)

Hypertension is one of the most common chronic health conditions in society today and has been called the silent killer because it usually has no symptoms. Fortunately hypertension is easily diagnosed and usually treatable.

Risks of hypertension

Heart attack   (High blood pressure can double or triple your risk)
Stroke   (High blood pressure can triple or quadruple your risk)
Kidney disease (Next to diabetes, this is the most common cause of kidney disease)
Vision problems

You are at increased risk of having high blood pressure if you are:

- Overweight
- A smoker
- Inactive
- African-American
- A person with a family history of hypertension

HOME SUGGESTIONS

1   If you are a smoker it is vital that you quit smoking.
2   If you are overweight, you need to reduce your weight. Studies show that if you lose as little as 10%, you begin to see an effect on your blood pressure.
3   If you are inactive you should gradually start to exercise. If you are otherwise healthy, you should aim for 30 to 40 minutes of daily aerobic exercise. This means that you are exercising at a level that makes you mildly short of breath and sweaty. See **EXERCISE** on page 185.
4   Maintain your intake of alcohol intake at a level of 2 drinks a day or less for men or 1.5 drinks a day or less for women.
5   Avoid decongestants and cough, cold and allergy medicines that have decongestants in them. If you are unsure, ask your pharmacist for help.
6   Learn relaxation/stress reduction techniques. If you have a stressful job, find one or two times during the day when you can escape to a place of temporary relaxation.
7   If you are hypertensive you should;
    - Reduce your salt intake in your diet. Do not add extra salt. Take the salt shaker off the table.
    - Do not miss doses of your medication.
    - Make sure you get adequate calcium and potassium in your diet.
    - Consider purchasing your own blood pressure monitor.

White coat hypertension and home blood pressure monitoring

Almost everyone's blood pressure goes up when they are in the doctor's office. For some the elevation is minimal but for others the temporary elevation is very significant. When you do proper measurements outside the doctor's office you add vital information that can help determine whether you need medication or not or how much medication you need to control your blood pressure. Excellent blood pressure monitors are available at your pharmacy and are very simple to use.

INFORMATION

Recommended Blood Pressure Targets of The Heart and Stroke Foundation

Category	Systolic/Diastolic
Optimal	120/80 or lower
Normal	120-129/80-84
High-Normal	130-139/85-89
High Blood Pressure	140/90 or higher
High Blood Pressure in people with Diabetes or kidney disease	130/80 or higher
High Blood Pressure with self/home Monitoring	135/85 or higher

What do the two numbers mean?

The pressure in your arteries is not constant. The top number represents the pressure when it peaks as the heart pumps blood into the system.The lower number represents the pressure that exists when it falls as the heart relaxes between beats. The top number is called your systolic pressure and the bottom number is called diastolic pressure. Both are important and need to be monitored to prevent conditions that can be a result of high pressure.

Sexually Transmitted Diseases

Sexually transmitted diseases (STDs) are diseases that can be passed to someone else by having sex with them. They are caused by both viruses and bacteria. Unfortunately many or most of the people who carry a disease do not know that they are infected.

Who is at risk?

Everyone who is sexually active with someone other than a STD-free, monogamous partner is at risk. The more sexual partners that you have, the higher your risk of infection. Activities that can transmit infection include: sexual intercourse, anal intercourse, genital to genital contact and oral sex. Sexual intercourse while using condoms reduces but does not eliminate the risk.

What to look for

- Sores or pain in the genital area (penis and inside or outside the vagina), anal area, or the mouth, tongue or throat if there has been oral sex
- Discharge from the vagina or penis
- Painful urination
- Warts around the genital area
- Flu like symptoms: fever, fatigue, sweats and body ache
- Swollen glands in the genital area
- Unusual infections
- Lower abdominal pain

If you have any of these symptoms or are simply concerned because of your sexual activity you should see your doctor.

How do you protect yourself?

First of all you must consider the risks of your sexual activity. The only way to be 100% safe is to not be sexually active. Other than that the safest alternative is to limit your sexual activity to a partner that you know is free of infection.

As you increase the number of your partners you greatly increase your risks. Remember the phrase, "When you have sex with someone you have sex with everyone they have had sex with." Combine this with the fact that many people who are infected are not aware of it and as a result do not feel any need to warn a partner or take precautions. You should also consider the increased risk of having sex with known prostitutes (male or female) and avoid casual sexual encounters. One is naive not to realize that when people are looking for sex it is not in their best interest to announce the fact that they have an STD. You must take care of yourself and not rely on your partner.

Condoms greatly decrease but do not eliminate your risk of an STD and should be used every time you have vaginal, anal or oral sex. The female condom is not as effective but is beneficial when a male condom will not be used or is not available. Some diseases can be spread just by the body contact in the genital area that is not covered by a condom. Condoms can break, even when used properly. Using spermicidal foams or jellies, designed to prevent pregnancy, may increase your risks of an STD due to the inflammation they may cause. It is vital that you follow the instructions for using a condom properly. Never reuse a condom.

The most common STDs are:

- **Herpes** (HSV or Herpes Simplex Virus)
- **Chlamydia** The most common preventable cause of female infertility
- **Human Papilloma Virus** (HPV) The cause of cervical cancer and genital warts
- **HIV** Can result in AIDS
- **Syphilis**
- **Gonorrhea**
- **Hepatitis B and C**

Visual Impairment and Eye Health

Most vision problems arise from the shape of your eyes. Sitting too close to the TV or reading under low light will not change your vision. You can't go blind by doing it too much, no matter what it is.

Near-sightedness or myopia means that one has difficulty focusing on objects further away. Far-sightedness or hyperopia means you have problems focusing on objects up close. Some vision problems may be permanently changed by reshaping the front of the eye with laser surgery.

It is very common for people to become less able to focus up close as they age. This is caused by a change in the lens of the eye. Reading glasses are commonly needed after age 45.

There are medical problems that may rob people of their vision slowly over time.

Glaucoma is a disease of increased pressure inside the eye. Treatments may include laser surgery and medication. Treating glaucoma before it causes vision loss is important. You can be tested for glaucoma in an eye exam.

Macular degeneration is a slow deterioration of the back of the eye called the retina. If the retina doesn't work your brain doesn't get the right information. There are therapies to slow macular degeneration. It is a common problem and can be diagnosed only with an examination.

Optomotrists and ophthalmologists are both trained to examine eyes and diagnose these common problems.

Eye safety

Remember you only have two eyes. You need to protect your eyes from the sun's dangerous ultra violet waves as much as your skin. Buy sunglasses that block UVA and UVB. It is money well spent. Pucks move fast and balls can make wild bounces so it is important to protect your eyes during sports. Wear CSA approved eye protection. It may be cool to play without eye protection, but eye patches have gone out of style.

Diabetes

Diabetes is a common disease and occurs when your pancreas does not produce enough insulin or your body does not use the insulin it does produce effectively. Insulin is released when the level of sugar in your blood rises, and enables your body to use or store the sugar. Without insulin, sugar levels rise and over time can cause serious damage.

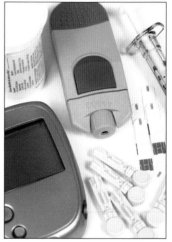

There are two types of diabetes:

Type 1. This condition develops when the pancreas stops producing insulin properly, so the person must inject insulin to replace the production. This can happen at any age but is most common in children and young adults.

Type 2. This is the most common form of diabetes. Type 2 diabetes develops in adults of any age and more frequently in the obese. Initially, type 2 diabetics have elevated blood sugars because their bodies no longer use insulin effectively. Eventually the pancreas may fail to produce enough insulin and the disorder worsens. Control of Type 2 diabetes initially involves diet control, weight loss and some oral medications. If unsuccessful or if the disease becomes more severe, patients may need to use insulin by injection.

Symptoms of an elevated blood sugar level include:

- Constant thirst
- Frequent urination
- Increased appetite
- Unusual fatigue
- Blurry vision
- Skin infections or slow healing wounds
- Recurring vaginitis or urinary tract infections
- Unexplained weight loss
- Erectile dysfunction

You are at risk of diabetes if you:

- Are over 45 years
- Are overweight
- Have a family history of diabetes
- Are of African-American, Hispanic, Native American or Asian American descent

Diabetes can cause

- Heart disease and stroke
- Nerve damage
- Kidney failure
- Blindness

Avoid diabetes or diabetic complications by:

- Eating a well-balanced diet, avoiding foods that are high in sugar or fat. If you are diabetic you should see a dietician and follow their advice.
- Maintaining a healthy weight.
- Exercising (see page 185).
- Quitting smoking.
- Checking your blood pressure and cholesterol.

If you are diabetic, you must monitor your blood sugars closely.

Index

INDEX

About the authors

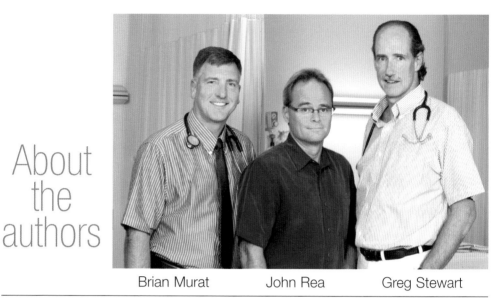

Brian Murat   John Rea   Greg Stewart

Greg Stewart MD., CCFP., is a Family Physician who lives in Huntsville, Ontario with his wife Charlene and their two sons. He received his Bachelor of Commerce degree from Mount Allison University and went on to complete Medical School at Memorial University in Newfoundland. His postgraduate training took place at Dalhousie University. In Huntsville his duties include being a staff physician in the Emergency Department and the Co-ordinator of Continuing Medical Education. He also conducts an annual medical conference for Family Physicians to which physicians have come from around the province and across the country. He enjoys primary care medicine and the patient education opportunities that it provides. This book has offered him an opportunity to reach out beyond his own practice population to give many others the same basic medical advice he gives his own patients.

Brian Murat MD., FRCPC., is a specialist in Internal Medicine and Gastroenterology. He completed his Medical Degree at Queen's University at Kingston in 1985. His postgraduate training included a general internship at St. Michael's Hospital in Toronto followed by a residency in Internal Medicine in Toronto. He returned to Queen's for his training in Gastroenterology. He now lives in Huntsville, Ontario with his wife, Ann and their three children. His practice includes both comprehensive Gastroenterology, as well as a variety of Emergency Internal Medicine experiences. His interest in public education stems from his personal experience in empowering patients with the knowledge of physiology and pathology resulting in much happier patients who learn to help manage their difficulties as part of a team. He believes that there is a large population of people who are thirsting for the tools to help themselves. This book is an attempt to supply those tools.

John Rea MD, CCFP(EM), FCFP. Dr. Rea completed his medical training in Ottawa, Ontario including his Family Medicine residency and Certificate of Special Competence in Emergency Medicine. He practised Emergency Medicine in Ottawa for two years before heading to Hunstville, Ontario to pursue his desire to practise comprehensive family medicine including Obstetrics and Emergency Medicine. He was Emergency Director for ten years. He has an interest in Medical Education and as a Clinical Instructor at the University of Ottawa he introduced the Family Medicine residency program to Huntsville. He continues teaching students as Associate Professor with the Northern Ontario School of Medicine. As an Executive Board Member for the Family Physicians Airway Group of Canada he has given lectures and workshops across Canada. He is the medical liaison for the Huntsville Respiratory Clinic. Interest in research has led to participation as an Investigator in several Primary Care studies and contribution to several Clinical Practise Guidelines and Family Medicine texts. He served two terms as the Georgian representative on the Board of the Ontario College of Family Physicians and enjoys consultant work for the Canadian Medical Protective Association. He enjoys the outdoors lifestyle in Muskoka with his wife and their four active children.